Life-Changing Praise for Airway is Life

I highly recommend this book to anyone that wants or needs to learn more about Sleep Disordered Breathing (SDB). As doctors we often speak in "Doctorese", a linguistic quagmire of technical jargon and polysyllabic utterances that can sound like a foreign language. "Doctorese" leaves patients feeling confused and frustrated at leaving with more questions than answers. If you have ever felt this way, this book was written for you.

In using a combination of simple language and the stories of real patients to explain these advanced concepts, Dr. Dassani has created something that has long been missing in our field, a text on Sleep Disordered Breathing that people without a medical degree can read, understand and even enjoy. When dealing with something as important as the subject of Sleep Disordered Breathing, the ability to communicate complex concepts and information in an easy to understand but also highly accurate way is invaluable. Dr. Dassani accomplishes this with aplomb.

—Christopher S. Hoffpauir, DDS

Practical wisdom to improve one of the most important areas of our life – sleep!

Dr. Dassani sheds new light on ways dentistry supports airway flow, proper breathing and restorative sleep. Breath is life, this is huge.

—Victoria Peterson, SsD
Productive Dentist Academy

Dr. Dassani's passion for saving lives shines through in everything she does. This book is remarkable in that it is not only extremely comprehensive, but it's written and organized in such a way that it is easy to understand for both professionals and for patients. It's a must read for anyone venturing on discovery about healthy sleep. Highly recommended.

—Amanda Sheehan, DDS

Airway is Life: Waking up to your family's sleep crisis is a compelling look at the multifaceted way sleep affects us. From ADHD to processing strong emotions to hormonal weight gain, healthy sleep and a healthy airway is critical for our families to live their best lives and true callings. Dr. Dassani is passionate about improving the lives of others through improved knowledge of sleep.

—Meghan Welden Darby, DMD

Whoever knew that breathing wasn't easy? Airway is Life sure is an eye opener that discloses daily events happening in our body that sets off alarms, to warn us about the distress going on, yet we turn a blind eye towards it and deem it normal. I love how this book reveals our body's little secrets happening under the cover of sleep. It teaches us everything we never knew about the relationship between sleep and airway, a healthy life and a sleep deprived life, an energetic day and a sluggish day, and why we behave the way we do. The different processes that take place to build our brain and clear a path for learning in our sleep. It seems like a good reason to change our sleeping habits because who wants to forget things, remain tired and have a lag in our motor skills. This is apparently just a few of the many things that happen in our body due to our compromised sleep and airway issues. The truth that shook my world was how weight loss was impeded by the lack of good sleep. Apnea appears to be the biggest causative agent to all our sleep troubles. Again, who knew breathing wasn't easy. Dr.Dassani's book is exquisitely laid out to identify the indicators of sleep apnea,which further helps us look into our health and wellness. It is a good easy read, flows well and enlightens our mind at the same time. Highly recommend this amazing book. A TRULY BRILLIANT MASTERPIECE!

—Linty John- Varghese, DDS

I have had the pleasure to read Airway is Life, beyond being very educational about sleep patterns and the way it affects our daily lives, it definitely conveys the importance of a true good night's rest. Reading about how much impact our sleep habits have on our health, daily patterns, and overall safety was certainly educational and informative. I feel very fortunate to have had the opportunity to learn about the "airway is life" through Dr. Dassani's new book. Personally, the Airway Is Life is a new form of maintaining an overall healthy and active life, it's definitely a practice that is so underutilized. I most definitely recommend reading Airway is Life

—Rebecca Streisfield

In this well researched book, Dr. Meghna Dassani helps both healthcare professionals and patients understand the importance of recognizing and treating sleep related disorders. Dr. Dassani provides clear explanations about the multiple interrelationships between lack of restorative sleep and multiple different physical and psychological conditions. The real-life examples of people whose health issues were resolved following treatment for sleep disordered breathing help connect the dots for physicians and dentists faced with patients who present with similar complaints. This book is an excellent learning tool and resource for laypeople and a must read for all healthcare professionals who want to improve the patient's quality of life.

—Kathryn Gilliam, RDH

Airway is life is a book I wish I would have gotten my hands on long before having children. Such valuable information that can change once life. My journey with questioning sleep issues began with my twelve-year-old son who was still wetting the bed at night. We tried no drinks after a certain time, diet change, and chiropractic care and nothing seemed to help. After much research I learned about obstructed airways and my son seemed to have all the symptoms. I immediately looked for a provider in my area. Expanding his airway was the missing piece. My other children are now also having their airway expanded so they too can experience the beauty of healthy sleep. I am grateful to have found Dr. Dassani as she has impacted our lives with her care and wealth of knowledge.

—Erika Gray

I have learned so much from this brilliant read about why my brain is wiped out at 5:00 p.m. after a busy day. I knew sleep was important, but now I know why it's crucial to grow, learn and retain. With Dr. Dassani's knowledge and ability to make logic and science accessible, lives can be changed. This is a must-read for all of us. It gives new weight to my mother's nighttime blessing: "Sleep tight, don't let the bed bugs bite."

—Anne Duffy

Airway is Life

WAKING UP TO YOUR FAMILY'S SLEEP CRISIS

MEGHNA DASSANI DMD

Copyright © 2021 by Meghna Dassani DMD

All rights reserved. No part of this publication may be reproduced, stored in a retrieval system, or transmitted, in any form or by any means, except as may be expressly permitted by the 1976 Copyright Act or by the copyright holder/publisher in writing.

ISBN: 978-1-7366589-1-8 (paperback)
ISBN: 978-1-7366589-0-1 (ebook)

Whilst every effort has been made to ensure that the information contained within this book is correct at the time of going to press, the author and publisher can take no responsibility for the errors or omissions contained within.

Book design by Wordzworth
Cover design by Alana Rodrigues

FOR MOM,
The woman I aspire to be some day.

Contents

Foreword　　　　　　　　　　　　　　　　　　　　　　　xi

Acknowledgments　　　　　　　　　　　　　　　　　　　xv

Introduction　　　　　　　　　　　　　　　　　　　　　xvii

PART 1	**IT ALL BEGINS WITH SLEEP**	**1**
Chapter 1	What is Sleep, Anyway?	3
Chapter 2	The Work of Sleep	13
PART 2	**WHEN SLEEP GOES WRONG**	**35**
Chapter 3	What Keeps Us Awake?	37
Chapter 4	Stolen Breath, Stolen Sleep	49
Chapter 5	The Sleepless Brain	69
Chapter 6	When Your Child Isn't Sleeping: Profiles of Sleep Disordered Breathing (SDB) in Children and Teens	91
Chapter 7	Adults Need Sleep Too—What it Looks Like When They Aren't Getting It	103
Chapter 8	Short on Sleep, Long on Problems— The Long-Term Consequences of Sleep Disordered Breathing	113

| PART 3 | GETTING HELP FOR SLEEP PROBLEMS | 129 |

Chapter 9   When You Suspect a Sleep Problem, What Comes Next?   131

Chapter 10   What Do All These Tests Mean and Will They Hurt?   147

Chapter 11   How We Fix Broken Sleep   159

Chapter 12   On Your Way To Better Sleep   187

Glossary of Sleep Science Terms   191

Further Reading   197

Sources   199

Foreword

We have all had the experience of meeting somebody for the first time and noticing something about them. Something different. Something unusual, almost as if they have a light or an energy. We can't always put our finger on it, but something inside us sees that *something* inside them. Such was the first interaction and meeting that I had with Dr. Meghna Dassani. Our relationship began, as so many others have, over the last few years, through mutual friends and an online connection. It has since morphed into a beautiful, personal, professional, and intellectual indulgence for me: collaborating with and advising her on her journey to spread her individual brand of magic into the world through her businesses. The kind of magic you are about to get a good dose of.

It didn't take long for me to start seeing what it was about her that resonated with me in that first meeting: vitality. It radiates from her. She is, as with the finest versions of my successful entrepreneurial clients, a living example of the very wisdom, philosophy, and medicine that she practices. She is a product of her product: healthy, vibrant, present, and giving.

We should all be so fortunate.

Yet, now we are, quite simply, as a reader of this book.

Airway is Life.

Contemplatists first acknowledged the existence of "air" over two thousand years ago. Experiments by Philo of Byzantium in the second century BCE were the first documented to identify the relationship between air and combustion. Leonardo da Vinci added to that work 1500 years later, with his own experimentation that displayed a further connection between air and respiration. Slowly, the possibility that "air" was, in fact, a catchall for a number of elements began to emerge.

It took another 100 years before the specific identification and naming of oxygen even arose in our awareness and language.

Early progress was slow in understanding oxygen's role and impact in the universe and in our lives. Such is the case with all frontiers of science—it's slow, messy work that we struggle to make sense of and connect to our own experience. In 1774 British clergyman Joseph Priestley was successful in isolating oxygen and set about testing its power and influence on plants, animals, fire, and even himself. He soon noticed a theme: all of these things appeared to thrive when they were exposed to it, including himself. Of his experience, he noted in his research diary, "The feeling of it to my lungs was not sensibly different from that of **common air**, but I fancied that my breast felt peculiarly light and easy for some time afterwards."

Science is the ongoing discovery of our prior ignorance. The true nature of things. Things we previously were so sure of, only to learn how little we actually understood. In that sense, what you are about to experience in the pages that lie ahead is pure science: a series of perspective-shifting insights and upgrades of all the things you thought you knew about your own health and that of your loved ones.

It is equally and deliberately a book that any non-scientist will immediately understand and resonate with from their own personal experience.

Just like Joseph Priestley.

Oxygen is the third most abundant element in the universe by mass. We are blind to its ubiquity and life-supporting role in our everyday lives.

By wonderful coincidence, humans spend approximately one-third of their lives asleep. Here too, we are blind to its ubiquity and life-supporting role in our everyday lives.

We are so quick to medicate ourselves, looking to "optimize" or "hack" our own health. We hop between new diets and exercise routines constantly searching for that new cool thing that will make a difference. We scrutinize labels, count calories, and measure our macros. We take supplements to help us sleep and caffeine to wake us up a few hours later. We spend a fortune on equipment that inevitably ends up in the basement, doing service as an overpriced coat hanger.

We toil away at our desks, hunched over for countless hours in an enormous gamble that joy and wellbeing will be waiting for us in the future. We'll sleep when we're dead, we say.

Vitality is always just one more pill or ten more pounds away.

Maybe.

Maybe not.

Perhaps the secrets to unlocking the health we so desperately seek, labor, and long for is hiding in plain sight. In the dark recesses of our cool bedroom and comfortable bed. In the hunched and stifling posture of your work desk. In the narrow, constricted palate of your permanently-distracted child. Perhaps it's hidden in the jokes about Grandpa's snoring and the lack of connection to his myriad health issues. The unspoken family concern about Mom's fading memory and focus. In our short attention spans and even shorter tempers.

Airway is Life.

It is connected to and supporting every single thing you do yet gets none of the attention it deserves. Until now. As you are about to learn, backed by a growing mountain of research and evidence, the quality of our airways is more connected to the quality of our lives than just about anything we could imagine. Prepare to be amazed at the patterns and issues you will discover in your own life and circles as you move so easily through the pages ahead.

Dr. Dassani has a magic that is changing lives. The world will soon beat a path to her door in search of it.

Yet here she is, coming to yours.

Sit back and allow her magic and wisdom to change yours, just as she has and does my own.

Alastair J. Macdonald

Acknowledgments

This book wouldn't have been possible without my patients that trusted me to help them breathe better and sleep better over the last ten years.

I'm immensely grateful to the amazing team I have the pleasure of working alongside every single day that gives their all to make sure our patients are well taken care of. Christina who keeps my world on track. Vanna who epitomizes sunshine every single day. Crystal and Erika who make everything I do seem so effortless.

What an indescribable pleasure it is to work with people who are genuinely interested in serving our patients and who are always eager to support and help test new ideas and ways of thinking.

I want to acknowledge Alastair Macdonald, who is not only my mentor and coach but has also become my family.

Sweta, my sister and partner in crime since we were little, has constantly encouraged me to "get that book out of my head."

I can't thank Chris Hoffpauir enough for being my unrelenting source of inspiration to challenge the status quo and change how dentists and the world understand sleep-disordered breathing.

I'm deeply indebted to Laura Moriarity for her wonderful editorial support and guidance.

Finally, a huge thank you to my parents, friends, and family that have believed in me and supported my dreams.

Last but not least, I owe an enormous debt of gratitude to my husband, Rahul, and my girls Nandini and Maadhvi for tolerating my incessant disappearances into my world of sleep-disordered breathing ... a family that makes both the journey and destination worthwhile.

Introduction

If you've picked up this book, you probably have a reason to learn more about sleep breathing. Maybe you, or someone in your house, snores. The noise is taking a toll on everyone's rest and health, and you're desperate for answers and solutions.

Maybe your physician or dentist gave you this book and suggested that you read it and see if anything sounds familiar. Could your blood pressure, weight gain, blood sugar, or pain issues be related to how you're sleeping? Could there be a way to address the underlying issue and save your life?

Or perhaps, your child is showing signs of ADHD, yet you're not convinced that stimulant drugs are the answer. What else can cause ADHD symptoms in a child? Could there be unresolved sleep issues?

Maybe you have a bedwetter or a mouth-breather in your family. Maybe someone is always tired and draggy, even after hours in bed. Maybe you feel like it's impossible to breathe when you're on your back.

Or maybe you're just curious. Why is everyone talking about OSA these days? Could it be worth it to get screened? Breathing machines like the CPAP are such a hassle. Are there other options for you and your kids, and what are those options?

Whatever your reason for picking up this book, I want to emphasize: *Airway is Life.* When your sleep breathing isn't working right, nothing else will work either.

I've spent years introducing my dental patients to sleep medicine and solving their problems through a combination of screenings, referrals, and treatments. I regularly work with multidisciplinary teams to get my patients' airways open so that they can get good, high-quality rest. I lecture internationally and even teach other dentists how to add sleep medicine to their practices.

I am passionate about making sure that people know about the importance of sleep. I want to connect people to the care they need so that they can get those airways open. I hope, after you finish this book, you'll understand the importance of sleep and sleep breathing and share what you've learned with your friends and family. Airway is life, and together, we can save the lives of the people we love.

PART 1

It All Begins with Sleep

"A soul submerged in sleep is hard at work and helps make something of the world."

—Heraclitus—

1

What is Sleep, Anyway?

*"O soothest Sleep! if so it please thee, close
In midst of this thine hymn my willing eyes"*

—John Keats—

Have you ever sat and watched someone sleep? Perhaps you woke up and looked at your spouse in the middle of the night. Maybe you held a sleeping infant in your arms for hours, looking down at them with love. Or perhaps you've been at the bedside of someone who was very sick or in pain and watched them finally let go enough to be able to sleep.

Sleep is weird when we watch other people do it. Sometimes, their faces and bodies are so still that we wonder if they're even alive. In our more paranoid moments, we may lean close or stick our hand near their face so we can see if they're still breathing. Sometimes, sleeping people might twitch or grimace. Small children may even have night terrors, where they're awake and flailing and screaming but not really **there**.

Sleep has interested, enticed, and confused philosophers and scientists since ancient times. Even today, sleep science is a fairly new medical field. We're finding out new things about sleep all the time. So, before we get into why our sleep breathing is so important, let's start with a little background on what we know about sleep—and what science has left to learn.

As we learn about sleep, I'll also weave in the stories of real people I've known and their sleeping issues. (Names and details have been slightly changed to provide anonymity.) You may recognize yourself in some of these people—their stories are important because so many people share them. If one of these stories strikes too close to home, please don't wait to finish the book. Make a sleep screening appointment today.

Sleep in History and Culture

In ancient times, people had no way to look inside the brain and see what was going on during sleep. Instead, they had to figure out for themselves what was happening, based on watching people who slept, the dreams that they themselves remembered, and seeing how people felt when they didn't sleep.

In many religious traditions, dreams were thought to have great significance. They were messages from deities giving warnings, advice, or predictions about the future. Sleep itself was a liminal state that is a doorway between two kinds of existence. For many, sleep represented a place in-between life and death. In fact, death itself was sometimes seen as a sort of perpetual sleep.

As science developed, philosophers and scientists began to examine sleep more closely. The Greek philosopher Aristotle suggested that dreams weren't sent from the outside, but instead something that came from our own consciousness. People began to test to see if sleepers were truly unconscious or if they could respond to outside events like a loud noise or a hand placed in a bowl of water.

Even in ancient times, doctors were convinced that sleep was necessary for good health and for recovery from illness. In ancient Egypt, doctors would give patients syrups made from poppies to help them sleep. In Medieval Europe, pharmacists would sell mixes of wine and herbs to help people sleep. Drugs designed to cause sleep became popular in the nineteenth century, as did the idea of a "rest cure," where a chronically ill person could go somewhere to rest, sleep, and hopefully heal. Doctors prescribed these sleep aids because they seemed to work, but they had no underlying science to describe how these chemicals made people sleep.

At the beginning of the twentieth century, sleep science was born. Scientists finally had the tools to see some of what was going on in the brain. In 1937, scientists first began using electroencephalogram (EEG) to study electrical patterns in the brain during sleep. This showed that the brain is active during all stages of sleep and that different parts of the brain are active at different stages. It also allowed scientists to test whether the brain responded to noises or smells when the body appeared not to. In 1957, the scientists Nathaniel Kleitman and William Dement described the five stages of sleep, further broken down into REM, or rapid eye movement, and NREM, non-rapid eye movement.

Scientists also learned about circadian rhythms. They began to understand that there were forces compelling people to sleep at certain times of the day and be awake at others. For most people, the time to sleep was at night, but for other people, it seemed like the night was a time to be awake and keep watch. When these people were in jobs that suited their schedules, all was well, but when we forced them to sleep and wake against their natural rhythms, they had trouble staying awake and alert. These rhythms weren't even stable across the lifespan. Scientists began realizing that at different points in our lives, we may be morning people, night people, or something in between and that it's mostly beyond our control.

New technology lets scientists learn more about what happens when people sleep and what happens when they don't. In 1965, a group of scientists discovered Obstructive Sleep Apnea (OSA) and showed that people who were sleepy during the day often had trouble breathing at night. They noticed that this lack of sleep seemed to trigger weight gain, high blood pressure, and other metabolic issues. In 1975, researchers at Stanford showed that patients with sleep breathing issues and high blood pressure improved after surgery that corrected breathing. In 1981, with the invention of the CPAP (Continuous Positive Airway Pressure), a device that forces air into the airways during sleep, entered the mainstream, we finally had the tools to both detect sleep problems, especially sleep breathing problems, and ways to correct those issues.

Doug's wife dragged him in to see me. She had heard from a friend about the wonders our sleep medicine practice had worked, and she was hoping we could help. Doug was sluggish and tired, and his wife, Mandy, had a hard edge to her. "He stops breathing when he sleeps," she explained. "All the time. So, I'm not sleeping either because I have to stay awake to poke him until he starts breathing again." Tears started rolling down Mandy's face. "I'm so, so tired, Doctor. But I can't afford to sleep. If I let myself go, he could die!"

The Stages of Sleep, and What the Brain Does During Them

Scientists study sleep in special labs. They have volunteers agree to sleep while hooked up to machines that measure their brain waves, heart rate, and breathing. Doesn't sound very comfortable or restful, does it? But these monitors let researchers see what the body and the brain are doing while people are asleep.

Before the EEG, most doctors assumed that during sleep, the brain was like a machine that had been turned off. The body kept going, albeit more slowly, and the mind was gone. Today, we know that the brain is active in all stages of sleep and that it's possible to track how someone is sleeping by looking at their brainwaves.

Stage 0: When You're Awake

When you're awake, your brain waves, heart rate, breathing, and body temperature are constantly in flux. You're looking around, responding to the world, speeding up and slowing down, and constantly changing. You're taking in and processing information, eating and processing food, and moving around constantly. The only constant is change.

NREM Stage 1: Drifting Off

After a long day, you finally have a chance to lay down. You sink into your pillow and close your eyes. Within a few minutes, your breathing and heart rate slow. Your body temperature begins to drop. Your brainwaves change too. They become lower voltage than your daytime signals, and their pattern begins to change.

In stage one, your thoughts become more random and confused. You stop understanding the conversations and sounds around you. If someone wakes you up, you may not remember having slept at all. In stage one, you may experience "sleep jerks," where you feel like you're falling or thrashing and jerk yourself awake.

Most people spend between one and seven minutes in this stage of light sleep. When an exhausted new parent takes catnaps where they drift off for a few minutes in the middle of work or chores, they're hitting this stage of sleep. After you've spent several minutes in stage one REM, your brainwaves change again, and you've entered stage two.

Stage 2 NREM: Light Sleep

In stage two NREM, your brainwaves change again. They start forming "sleep spindles." If someone wakes you during stage two, you've only been in a light sleep. You can wake up and feel refreshed even though you haven't completed a complete sleep cycle. Many "power naps" take advantage of a short period of stage two sleep.

You'll remain in this stage for ten to twenty-five minutes. Slowly, the sleep spindles will become fewer, and the brain waves take on the slow, rhythmic patterns that mean that you've slipped into a deeper sleep.

Stages 3 and 4 NREM: Deep Sleep

Some scientists distinguish between stage three and stage four NREM, while others say that they're both parts of the same deep sleep. During these stages, a healthy person experiences slow, regular breathing, a slow heart rate, and synchronized, slow delta brain waves. This is the sleep you need to feel really and truly rested.

If you're a parent, you've probably seen a baby or child in a deep sleep. This is when they go limp. You can lift their arm, and it just falls back into place. You can move them around from a car to a bed, and they never even stir. Deeply sleeping adults can be hard to wake too, but their brains are still open to environmental stimulus. Researchers have found that during brief periods during each brain wave, the brain can respond to outside noises. So, even when you are deeply asleep, you can still hear the strange crash outside, the crying child, or the smoke alarm. Your brain is designed to keep you safe, even when you're sleeping.

This stage usually lasts from twenty to forty minutes. It ends with a return to stage two for five to ten minutes. After revisiting stage two, you don't return to stage one. Instead, you enter a state called REM.

REM: The Dreaming State

In REM, or rapid eye movement, sleep, your brain is as active as when you're awake. Sometimes it's even more active. Your eyes move rapidly, but the rest of your body experiences a kind of paralysis, so you won't move around and hurt yourself while you are dreaming. The rational centers of your brain are suppressed, but your emotional centers are running the show. The amount of time you spend in REM depends on the sleep cycle you're in. At the beginning of the night, your periods of REM are very short. Then, as the night goes on and you complete more sleep cycles, you spend more and more time in REM.

Sleep Cycles

Your brain moves between stage two, deep sleep, and REM sleep, all night long. Over the course of a good night's sleep, you'll spend about half the time in stage two. In each ninety-minute period, you'll experience stage two, stages three and four, and REM sleep. About four hours into your sleep, you may wake up and briefly move around, use the bathroom, or get a drink of water. Then you'll start back at stage one and begin again.

STAGES
OF **SLEEP**

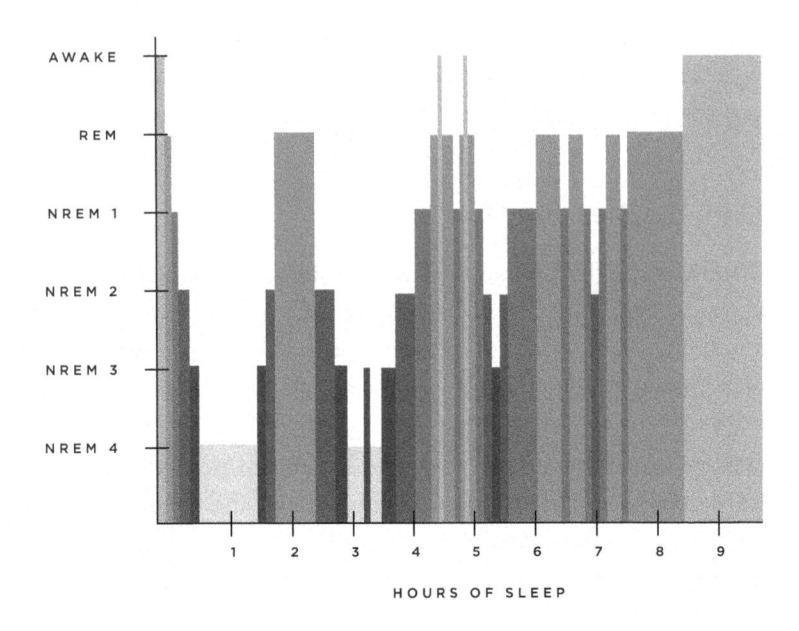

Figure 1. A Hypnogram is a graph that shows how a specific person cycles through sleep stages over the course of a night. Each person's hypnogram is unique to them. This is a sample hypnogram for a healthy adult.

Sleep cycles can be disrupted by insomnia, sleep breathing issues, or outside influences (like an infant who wakes you up every two hours). The cycles are constant, but the number of cycles varies by culture. For instance, some cultures sleep less at night but take a long afternoon nap. But individual sleep cycles seem to be similar across times and places. Sleep, and moving between light sleep, deep sleep, and dreams are an essential part of being human.

Now that you know what we can measure about sleep, it's time to find out what we think sleep does for the body.

The Take-Aways

- Sleep science is a young field. It really only began about seventy-five years ago, and we're discovering new things all the time
- Your sleep cycles repeat several times in a night because your body and brain have a lot of work to do.
- The EEG lets scientists see what's happening in your brain while you sleep, but you can learn a little about sleep by watching another person, or even a pet, sleep.

Try This

Watch another person or a pet sleep, and see if you can spot the move from stage two NREM to stage three and four NREM or from stage two NREM to REM. What do you notice?

Things to Think About

- Why did you decide to pick up this book?
- Who do you know who seems to need more sleep?
- Is there anyone you're going to share fun facts and information with as you read? Who?

2

The Work of Sleep

"A good laugh and a long sleep are the two best cures for anything."

—Irish Proverb—

We spend about a third of our lives sleeping, so it better be doing something, right? Otherwise, instead of teaching you how to make your sleep better, this book should be teaching you how to go without sleep!

Don't fear. Sleep is incredibly important for our bodies. In fact, the work of sleep is almost more important than the work we do while awake.

Without sleep, we lose our ability to learn, our ability to remember, our ability to work, to move, to digest. In fact, without the work of sleep, we lose our very selves. In this chapter, we're going to dig deep into the work of sleep and what each stage of sleep does for our minds and bodies. By the end, I hope you agree that healthy sleep is the key to a healthy life.

Experimenting on Sleepers: You Don't Know What You've Got 'Til It's Gone

Have you ever had to function on minimal sleep? Maybe you were up all night with a croupy baby but still had to go to work and care for your other kids the next day. Maybe you were a student, studying for exams or working hard to meet a deadline. Perhaps you were simply up worrying, thinking about things gone wrong, and unable to quiet your mind or body. Or maybe, you just were having so much fun you stayed up until near dawn.

How did you feel the next day?

If you're like most people, you probably felt fuzzy-headed, maybe a little sick. You may have had a burst of energy and then crashed. As the hours went on, you started nodding off, jerking awake, and trying all sorts of things to keep going. When the day ended, and you could finally go to bed, it was a sweet, sweet relief. Finally, you were where you needed to be. For researchers, it's not enough to know how we feel when we don't sleep. They also want to know why we feel that way and whether skipping different stages of sleep affects how we feel and act in different ways.

They're limited in the type of research they can do. You can't just keep a person up indefinitely and see what happens. They die. So, instead, they devise clever experiments where they have healthy college students miss out on sleep in different ways and then see what happens to people when you deprive them of all or some of their sleep.

By looking at how our minds and bodies fall apart when we don't sleep, the researchers have figured out at least some of the ways sleep keeps us together. However, sleep research is still a young field. They're discovering more about how sleep regulates the mind and body all the time.

Sleep and Hormones

When you think of hormones, you probably think of puberty. We talk a lot about hormonal teens and how hormones make them less predictable, more emotional, and generally hard to live with or teach. It's true; teen hormones can be a crazy rollercoaster. But everyone has hormones, all of the time. Currently, we've identified about fifty hormones in the human body, and researchers identify new hormones every few years.

Hormones are the equivalent of emails that cells in one part of the body send to other parts. They tell different organs how to react to changes in your environment. For instance, insulin is a hormone that regulates blood sugar. (It's one of SIXTEEN that control blood sugar regulation.) It's released from the pancreas when blood sugar rises, and it tells the cells in other parts of the body to start taking sugar out of the blood and either store it or use it to make energy. Insulin doesn't move the sugar out of the blood—different chemicals do that. But it tells the cells, "Sugar is coming; let it in."

Each of the hormones in your body sends different messages. And these hormones work day and night. Sleeping changes which hormones are being produced and how various cells react. Without this part of your daily cycle, your hormones will go haywire (even worse than they do in teenagers), your organs won't function correctly, and you'll get very sick very quickly.

So, what are the biggest ways sleep changes your hormones, and why do they matter?

Growth Hormone

A toddler is suddenly very hungry and very tired. The normally perky kid has been sleeping all the time for the last two days. Young parents wonder if their baby is sick. He doesn't have a fever, after all. Grandma volunteers, "I bet he's going through a growth spurt!" And, after a few days, the kid is bigger, and suddenly, his shoes no longer fit. What happened here?

Growth hormone, which tells cells to divide and heal, is released during sleep, and especially during the slow-wave sleep early in the night. This is the mechanism behind restorative sleep. During deep sleep, the body releases growth hormone, and new cells are made while old cells are repaired. So, kids with a lot of growing to do, need to do a lot of sleeping, and they sleep more when they're growing more.

What about adults? Well, we don't need to grow, but we need growth hormone to repair our damaged tissue. All-day long, our body endures wear and tear. During slow-wave sleep, the anterior pituitary gland releases growth hormone. The hormone circulates with our blood and helps our body:

- Keep blood sugar level as we sleep
- Repair damaged cells or encourage cell replication
- Break down fat
- Build new muscle

These are all essential functions if we want to wake rested, healed, and full of energy to face the day.

Cortisol

Cortisol is a get-up-and-go hormone. It's released by the adrenal gland and regulates many body functions throughout the day. Our circadian rhythms influence it, and it tends to be higher in the morning and lower at bedtime.

Cortisol is also a stress hormone. When we're in danger, it triggers the physical changes associated with "fight or flight." It raises our blood sugar so that cells have the energy they need for a quick escape or for difficult thinking. It suppresses "non-essential" functions, like certain immune reactions. It also lets us feel afraid and anxious, which can be important in a life or death situation. However, there's a problem, especially in today's world.

For a lot of us, especially adults, we experience low levels of "fight or flight" throughout the day. We're stressed out by work and health and money and news and life, and our body keeps us at the ready in case the slow-moving disasters become quick-moving ones. This is a huge strain on all of our body systems. Over time, this stress hormone means that we get sick more often, with a spiral of secondary effects. It causes us to gain weight. We're more nervous and can't interact with our communities as much. Everything starts falling apart under the constant, low-level exposure to excess cortisol.

So what does this have to do with sleep?

When we sleep, cortisol levels are suppressed. We get a break from the constant stress. Every cell in our body gets a break. Sleep gives us a chance to reset in a stress-free environment and protects our bodies and our immune system from the effects of daytime stress.

Ghrelin

Ghrelin is the hormone that regulates our appetite. It's produced in the stomach and surges when we fast or right before we eat. It's what makes us hungry. It also encourages our body to store calories as fat. During the day, the amount of ghrelin in our system decreases when we eat. Carbs and protein decrease it faster than fats do, which is why certain foods take the edge of hunger quickly.

When a teenager sits down and eats a gigantic sandwich, that's in response to ghrelin.

Ghrelin also stimulates the release of growth hormone. It tells the body, "Prepare to use all the nutrition that is coming your way!" When people diet or fast, their levels go up because the body is signaling it wants food. It's why it can be so hard to lose weight and also why some people prefer high protein diets when they're interested in weight loss.

So, what does sleep have to do with ghrelin? It suppresses it! To get a good night's sleep, we need to go eight to ten hours without eating anything. Our body and brain are hard at work, but it's work that needs to happen in bed. We can't be getting up to wander around and eat every few hours.

In a healthy person, sleep prevents hunger signals. An exception is when someone isn't getting enough calories. They may be too hungry to sleep for long because they're not eating enough to control ghrelin levels. Then they'll sleep a little and then wake up to forage for food—which is why midnight snacks are a danger to dieters.

Finally, if you don't sleep, you don't get the suppression effect. Instead, your body continues to release ghrelin, and demand food, at regular intervals, which is one reason why college kids pulling all-nighters get hungry.

Leptin

Leptin is another hormone that controls food intake, weight gain, and metabolism. The difference is that while ghrelin controls these things meal to meal, leptin controls them over a longer time period.

Living things tend to be in a state called *homeostasis*. (That's Greek for "staying the same.") It's not healthy to wildly swing between extremes. Your weight, body temperature, metabolism, and activity levels all tend to stay pretty level, and when they don't, it's because you're sick. Leptin is one of the hormones that regulate homeostasis.

Leptin is released by the fat cells, and it tells your body how many calories to take in and how fast to burn them. When your leptin is low, you eat more food, burn fewer calories, and gain weight. When it's high, you eat less, burn more calories, and lose weight.

Sleep makes your leptin levels rise. You're not hungry overnight, and your body has permission to burn the calories it needs to do the work of sleep.

What Happens to Hormones When You Don't Sleep?

Becky came to my practice because she was grinding her teeth at night and wanted to stop. When we took her medical history, we found out that she snored and felt tired and fuzzy all the time. She had recently been diagnosed with high blood pressure and pre-diabetes, and her bloodwork was always off. She was gaining weight and just couldn't stop. It seemed like nothing she did affected her health in any positive way. She was ready to give up. Becky also had a history of hypothyroidism and wondered if TSH was responsible for all of her issues, but her doctor kept insisting her numbers there looked fine, and there must be something else going on, or that the answer was more diet and exercise, even though she was already eating a healthy diet and exercising

What she didn't realize was that she was showing all the signs of someone whose hormones were out of whack from a lack of good, restful sleep. We got her a referral for a sleep study, and it turned out she had OSA. Once the OSA was treated, the diet and exercise could actually do their work, and Becky got her health back.

Think about the times when people "naturally" lose sleep. During illness, natural disasters, family problems, wars, or famines, people sleep less. They're awake more because it's not safe to sleep, and their bodies hold themselves at ready in case they need to flee or fight off a threat. This makes sense. Sleep is a vulnerable time. When we can't afford to be unconscious, we can't afford to sleep.

So, what happens when we intentionally deprive ourselves of sleep for other reasons, like studying, working, playing video games, or binge-watching a favorite show?

The processes that control our hormones aren't fine-tuned enough to track *why* we're not sleeping. If we aren't getting a full night's sleep, our body goes into disaster preparation mode. Instead of healing and growing, we're focused on preparing for an imminent disaster.

Cortisol rises, raising our blood sugar, so we have energy handy. Growth hormone levels drop. Now's not the time to rest and repair. It's time to run. Ghrelin rises. Better eat now because who knows when you'll be able to eat again? You may be fleeing armies or scavenging for scarce resources soon, after all. Leptin drops. It's time to eat more and to burn calories more slowly. There may be a long journey ahead.

These changes make sense when you look at the long sweep of human history. But what happens when you're living a comfortable, twenty-first-century life and only skipping on sleep because you wanted to see what your favorite characters are up to?

We'll go into this more later, but for now, I want to leave you with a few thoughts:

- If good sleep is necessary to keep my body healthy and my hormones balanced, what am I doing to myself when I don't get a good night's rest?
- What are my family members doing to themselves?

- If I could change one thing about our sleep habits right now, what would it be?

This is just the work of sleep on your hormones, but there's another huge task that sleep completes each night. Sleep works on our brains and helps make us the people we are.

HORMONE	WITH SLEEP	WITHOUT SLEEP
Human Growth Hormone (HGH)	Increases Sends signal to body to grow and heal	No increase Body continues to take damage because you are awake Repair process doesn't occur Over time, more and more damage, harder to reverse
Cortisol (Stress Hormone)	Decreases Break from stress Rest from fight or flight Reduced damage and inflammation and pain	Doesn't decrease, may increase More stress More time in fight or flight More inflammation More damage to every system of your body
Ghrelin (Hunger Hormone)	Decreases You don't crave food while you sleep You do burn calories in	Continues to increase at intervals Get hungry every few hours Eat extra meals and calories Weight gain
Leptin (Satiety Hormone)	Increases You feel full and satisfied Your body is told it's OK to use calories	Decreases You crave food Your body tries to store more calories as fat Your body burns fewer calories, to conserve fat Weight Gain

How Sleep Builds Our Brains

Mike's mom was at her wit's end. Her 10-year-old son was struggling on multiple fronts at school.

He was diagnosed with dyslexia, but interventions didn't seem to be helping, and he kept falling further and further behind. He couldn't focus on his work. He wasn't able to memorize information, he seemed to have trouble processing when people talked to him, and his emotions were all up and down and all over the place.

As a result, he was always in trouble and was starting to think of himself as a "bad kid." After a screening, we sent him for an evaluation with the ENT. He had a tonsillectomy and adenectomy and got treatment for previously undiagnosed sinus and allergy issues.

Suddenly, he was a different kid. He was still dyslexic, of course, but he was finally making progress because his sleep improved, and he could actually learn. His moods leveled out, and so he was in trouble less and could handle frustration. He started being able to get along with peers, and for the first time in his life, Mike enjoyed school. He had never been a "bad kid." He'd been a sleep-deprived kid, and he was finally getting the rest he needed to learn and grow.

Sleep gives our body a chance to rest and recuperate from the day, but it doesn't mean that we're not doing anything. We burn about 82% of the calories burned in an hour watching TV in an hour of sleep. How can that be when we're not doing anything? Well, not only do our baseline metabolic activities continue, but our brains are actually hard at work.

Sleep isn't a break from brain activity. Instead, it's a shift in kinds of brain activity. During the day, we're constantly taking in information and learning new things about our environments, even if we're no longer students. We're seeing, hearing, smelling, touching, and tasting all sorts of things. We're moving—sometimes in familiar ways, but often in new ways. We're constantly interacting with other people, either in person or online or even through our televisions. All-day long, we're filling up our short memory with all of these facts, details, and impressions.

So, how can we constantly be interacting and learning without breaking down? We sleep! When we sleep, our brain shifts from a focus on collecting information to a focus on processing information. While we process little bits here and there during the day, nighttime is when the real work gets done.

Sleep does so many things for the mind:

- It makes it possible to learn new things.
- It stores new knowledge.
- It helps you practice motor skills.
- It helps you forget unimportant details.
- It helps process strong emotions.
- It rewires the brain when necessary due to growth, injury, or new skills.
- It helps us solve difficult problems.
- It makes us more creative.

How much time your brain spends in each activity changes as you grow. However, at every stage of life, sleep is essential for brain function.

Building the Brain before Birth and During Infancy

Sleep is so important that humans begin sleeping at around twenty-three weeks gestational age, right as they start a period of very fast brain growth and development. (Twenty-three weeks is also around the age that high-level NICUs can treat a premature baby.) In the womb, sleep is classified differently than in the sleep lab. Until the very end of pregnancy, the baby will sleep about twenty-four hours a day, with six hours of NREM sleep, six hours of REM sleep, and twelve hours of another stage that scientists haven't clearly defined yet. This is a time of rapid brain growth. The brain is creating and connecting neurons and wiring itself for the massive amount of learning that happens from the moment of birth.

For a full-term infant, the last two weeks before birth see a shift. The baby is still asleep most of the time but starts getting nine to twelve hours a day of REM sleep as the process of connecting neurons goes into overdrive. Does the amount of REM matter to such a small person? Yes!

Studies of preemies have found that babies who get more REM sleep are healthier. They spend more time growing and eating, less time crying, and more time focused and alert. Six months down the road, babies who get less REM sleep in the NICU have more neurological problems. It's unclear whether this is causation (lack of REM causes neurological problems) or correlation (babies with neurological problems also have dysfunctional REM sleep), but it's certain that the work done in REM sleep is important for long-term brain development.

Scientists have done experiments where they disrupt only the REM sleep of a group of newborn rats and then compare them to their peers. In these cases, the rats who undergo a few weeks of REM sleep disruption at a young age have brains that are wired in weird ways and grow up to be isolated, anti-social adult rats. So, even at very young ages, healthy, uninterrupted sleep with periods for REM matters to the brain.

Sleep Clears a Path to Learning

Have you ever had to do a task that was difficult, new, and took a lot of thinking? Your brain probably felt "fried" afterward. You were done with heavy thinking for the day and could only do mindless things. But then you woke up the next morning ready to tackle mentally challenging things again. What happened?

When you think hard, you learn new things. The part of your brain called the hypothalamus stores this new knowledge. But there's a problem. Your hypothalamus is sort of like the entryway of your brain. New information comes in the door and gets dropped there, just like your family drops mail and coats and backpacks and groceries. After a while, it gets cluttered. There's no room for new things until the old stuff has been examined, sorted, and either thrown out or stored in the proper place.

In sleep, the brain "cleans out" the hypothalamus and moves the new information to permanent storage. Waves of electricity pulse across the brain, and as this happens, new memories get moved to the appropriate parts of the brain. Facts, motor skills, things you've seen and need to recognize later, and social interactions all get moved to places where you can find them later.

This is like when you hang the coats in the closet, move the groceries to the refrigerator, sort the mail and put the bills on the desk, and put the backpacks back on their hooks after going through them to make sure there were no report cards or permission slips. After your work is done, your house is organized, and your front hall is clean and ready to start the new day. When your brain does work during sleep, the hypothalamus is cleaned out and ready to go, too.

If you don't get enough good sleep, and especially NREM sleep, the hypothalamus doesn't get totally cleaned out. You can't learn new things, and you're stuck.

This is also why people who are learning a lot very quickly often need naps. Have you ever watched a baby in an interesting and engaging environment, like a walk around the neighborhood? For a while, they're focused and busy, learning all they can about their environment. Trees, ducks, cars, dogs, they're all so interesting! But then suddenly, the kid is out like a light. They sleep for a while, wake up happy, and are interested again. What happened?

The baby's hypothalamus was full to the brim with new experiences and ideas, and they needed a nap to clear it out. After the nap, they're awake and ready to learn more. Researchers have seen a similar "nap effect" with college students. A group allowed to nap after learning new material was able to learn and retain more after the nap than a group that wasn't permitted a nap.

Since sleep clears the way for new learning, it makes sense to make good, uninterrupted sleep a priority, especially for people who go to school or have mentally taxing jobs. If we want people ready to take on new challenges every day, we need to make sure they slept the night before.

Sleep Stores New Knowledge for Easy Recall

Sleep is also important once you've learned things. While your brain is cleaning out that entryway, it's also processing and sorting the information it finds, just like you sort things in your house for storage. Holiday decorations go to the garage, out of season clothes to the attic, gardening tools to the shed. You don't look for a rake in the attic, and you don't expect to find the lights in the shed. Except, sometimes, if you don't have enough time to sort as you put things away, they may end up in the wrong places. And then, they either get permanently lost, or they're harder to find.

This can happen with insufficient sleep, as well. Studies done on elderly people find that those who have interrupted sleep have impaired memory a full decade before people who sleep well. Those forgotten appointments or errands can be a sign that you're not getting enough sleep to put new information where you need it to be. These things are literally slipping your mind because you need deep, uninterrupted sleep to store them properly.

This affects children too. For instance, in studies of kids with dyslexia, the children who have more sleep spindles, a feature of uninterrupted NREM stages two, three, and four sleep, are better readers than the children who don't have as many sleep spindles. This makes sense because a "hack" many dyslexics use in learning to read is memorizing the appearance of whole words to make up for the lack of phonics processing. The more whole words a dyslexic can memorize, the better they can read. And sleep is essential for transferring these new memorized words to the appropriate part of the brain.

Sleep can't cure dyslexia, but a lack of sleep can make it impossible for a child to develop coping mechanisms for working around their processing disorder.

Sleep Helps the Brain Learn New Muscle Skills

Think about all the things you can do almost without thinking. Walking, riding a bike, driving, writing with a pen or pencil, typing, playing an instrument—these are all things adults do without thinking about the discrete steps that go into every motion. But they're incredibly complex activities. And, at one time in your life, they were hard, they were new skills, and you had to concentrate while you did them.

When we talk about these things that become automatic, we like to talk about "muscle memory." But really, your muscles can't think or remember. They're moving in these familiar patterns because of signals from your brain. And your brain has practiced and remembered these patterns for so long that you no longer have to try and recall them.

You see a word and type it. You pluck out a familiar song on the piano. You sign your name on a paper. You drive to work and sing along with the radio. You walk around the block, stop to chat with a neighbor, and start walking again. Much of your day is easy and automatic, and you have sleep to thank for it.

When you've learned a new motor skill, the brain rehearses it during sleep. EEGs of sleepers who have learned new motor skills have activity in the motor cortex of the brain, the part responsible for movement. This means that the brain is running through the motions again and again, even as the body lies motionless.

Researchers have found that this activity happens most in the last two hours of an eight-hour stretch of sleep. It's not enough to practice a lot during the day. People learning new motor skills need to practice during the day *and then get a full eight hours of sleep after their practice.* Athletes who make sure to sleep a full night perform better and have fewer injuries than athletes who stint on sleep. Musicians who sleep a full night learn pieces faster and play better. If you want your children to learn to ride a bike sooner, to type and write better, and to be less clumsy, perhaps you should ensure that they get enough sleep.

The fact that motor memory happens at the end of sleep also has an important bearing on teen safety. Our teens are learning to drive, which means they have to quickly learn a host of new motor skills. Gas and breaks, steering, turn signals, and driving routes are very complicated. Just pulling out of a parking space uses so many muscle motions! When our teens are shortchanged on sleep, they're missing out on the brain activity necessary to make them better drivers. They're more at risk for deadly accidents, or at least fender benders.

This need for those last two hours of sleep may also explain why the elderly are so prone to fall injuries. As people age, they often have trouble staying asleep as long. If they're not getting a full eight hours, their brain isn't practicing motor skills as much, and that can lead to increased clumsiness. With frailer bodies, falls are more dangerous and can lead to painful injuries that cut sleep time even more. Lack of sufficient sleep is dangerous.

Sleep Helps Us Forget Unimportant Details

When your brain stores memories for easy access in sleep, it also performs another important job. It forgets things. You take in information all day. Some of it is important, like the dosing schedule for a new medicine or an article about when your street is finally going to be repaired. But a lot of information isn't worth remembering.

What did the car in front of you at the drive-through look like? Unless you got into an accident, you probably don't remember. How many pieces of junk mail did you get, and what was the price of that shirt you have no intention of buying? Who needs *that* sort of information cluttering up their thinking?

By making important information easy to access and erasing the useless stuff, sleep helps you think more quickly and focus on the task in front of you. The old information isn't erased right away, though, which means there's a window of a few days where you can choose to make sure information stays put. How?

- **Repetition.** If you need a fact over and over, your sleeping brain is more likely to put it where you can access it quickly.

- **The first time something happens.** New events are remembered more than repeats. So you might remember the first time you met someone with perfect clarity and some of the most recent meetings, but the middle might be a little fuzzy.

- **Unusual things.** We go through a lot of our lives looking for patterns and encountering familiar things. So when something is weird, it sticks out, and our brain hangs on to it.

- **Very emotional events.** Psychologically healthy people only feel strong emotion about important things, so strong emotion tags a memory as "important."
- **Cause and effect.** Your brain remembers things that have a strong cause and effect link because those are important memories. Things like "If I drive seventy-five on this road, I will get pulled over" are important to remember.

Do you have something you most certainly do *not* want to forget? Try using one of these "reasons for remembering" to hang onto it. Most of what you encounter in the day won't have one of these "important memory tags," and so within a few days, the memory will degrade until you can't remember whether it was a white SUV or a red coupe in front of you at that stoplight last week. You're just sure it wasn't a horse and buggy because *that* would have been worth remembering.

Sleep Helps You Process Strong Emotions

One of the most important purposes of REM sleep is the processing of emotions and social cues. It's especially important for events that trigger strong, unpleasant emotions. REM sleep allows people to work through feelings in dreams. Dreams won't exactly mimic daily life, but they have the same emotions. For instance, if you're really stressed about work, you might have a dream where you're back in high school, can't find your locker, and have to take an exam in a class you never attended. Your dreams help your brain deal with feelings of being in over your head, so you can face the next day a little less stressed and with a few more coping skills.

Dreams also help us process social interactions. In fact, when someone is deprived of REM sleep, they start losing their ability to interact with people in their daily lives. Their emotions are up and down, they miss important social cues, and they feel more anxious and interpret more people as hostile.

When an event is especially stressful, it may take more than one night of REM sleep to process it. Your dreams will come back to the strong emotion again and again until you've worked through the event and made it a part of who you are. REM sleep lets us live through the hard parts of life and yet continue to function.

So, what about post-traumatic stress disorder (PTSD)? Some studies have shown that people with PTSD have too much of a hormone that suppresses REM sleep. They can't process the event and their emotions in their sleep, so it starts creeping into their day, in the form of flashbacks. In one study, patients who received a drug that restored REM sleep were cured of PTSD. Their brains could finally do the work of processing emotions, and they were able to work through events and begin to function again.

If you recall, the time spent in REM per sleep cycle increases the closer you get to morning. That means that people who have to wake up earlier than their natural preference are missing out on emotional processing time. Could this be one reason our teens are so emotional? They're at an age of big feelings, but they rarely get enough REM time to process them.

Sleep Rewires the Brain

Have you ever noticed how kids get sleepier before a major developmental milestone? Sleep, and especially REM sleep, helps change how the brain is structured. At the end of pregnancy, brain growth goes into overdrive during REM sleep. Brains grow at an incredible rate until about age two, and most of this growth happens during REM sleep. Then, the pruning begins. REM sleep helps the brain eliminate unneeded connections and strengthen important ones. It makes thinking more efficient. Later, in the late tweens and early teens, REM helps the brain specialize.

We call this neuroplasticity. The brain can rewire itself to help people succeed. So, if a teen is doing a lot of math, the brain will strengthen math connections in preparation for adulthood. If a teen is an athlete, those connections get stronger during REM sleep. (This tendency to specialize does have a downside. If a teen is engaging in addictive behaviors, the brain will specialize in seeking out the addiction. This is one reason to remind your teens and tweens to focus on the right sorts of activities. The pruning going on in their teens helps set them up for life.)

Scientists have done experiments depriving adolescent animals of REM sleep. (They can't do these experiments on humans—the potential to completely ruin lives is too strong.) Rats deprived of REM sleep as "teens" grow up to be socially isolated and nervous. Other animals deprived of REM sleep at key developmental points are less able to learn new things as adults.

When an adult is deprived of REM sleep for a short time, they bounce back. But when our children and teens miss out on this sleep, it's gone. There is development and growth and specialization that never gets to happen.

The other time that sleep literally rewires the brain and creates new pathways is after an injury like an accident or a stroke. Over time, stroke victims can work with therapists and regain the functions they lost. What's happening is that, in sleep, the brain learns to reroute around the damaged areas to restore ability. After a stroke, a person's brain is not functioning exactly as it did beforehand, but REM rewires and reconnects so that they can recover.

Sleep Helps Us Solve Difficult Problems and Gives us Creativity

Have you ever had a problem and been told to "sleep on it and see what you think in the morning?" Did you wake up with a new outlook, a flash of inspiration, or a brilliant solution? If you did, thank REM sleep.

Scientists have done experiments where they give a group of college students tough problems to solve and then test them on their solutions after several hours have passed. Students who have REM sleep between seeing the problems and solving them can successfully solve more problems than the students who don't. The way REM sleep processes our experiences lets us make new connections and awake with new information about them.

While NREM sleep can strengthen memories and improve skills, during REM the brain combines bits of information and memories in new ways. This can spark new ideas and new solutions to old problems. This is why many scientists, mathematicians, musicians, and writers like to sleep with paper and pen by the bed. Many times, those first thoughts of the morning are important.

What does that mean for someone who never sleeps well enough for REM sleep? They're going to have a harder time with new problems. They're not going to be able to look at them from new angles and come up with solutions. They're going to be stuck.

If you don't want your family members to be stuck, you want to make sure they're getting good sleep.

Now that you appreciate how important sleep is, it's time to learn what happens when people can't get enough sleep and how to tell if someone you love may have sleep issues that are affecting their mental and physical health.

The Take-Aways

- We learn what sleep does for the brain and body by seeing what happens when we take it away.
- Sleep regulates your hormones and tells your body to heal after a busy day.

- Without sleep, metabolism is dysregulated—hello, weight gain, T2D, and cardiovascular issues!
- You need sleep to remember things and to learn how to do new things.
- Sleep is what gives you emotional control. You need it to be happy, social, and productive.

Try This

Make sleep a family priority for ONE NIGHT. Get ready for bed nine hours before you need to wake up. Turn off screens for two hours before that. How does it feel to wake up the next morning? How does your family feel different? Is there a way to start making sleep a priority at least one or two nights a week?

Things to Think About

- How much sleep do you normally get? Is it more than seven hours a night? Do you feel like you're getting enough?
- How is your emotional control? Can you make yourself do boring things? Can you handle setbacks cheerfully? Do you wish your emotional control was better?
- How quickly do you learn new things? Has learning gotten harder as you've aged? Have you tried sleeping more to help you learn more quickly?
- Does your partner or child have signs that they may not be getting enough high quality sleep? How can you help them make sleep a priority?

PART 2

When Sleep Goes Wrong

*"Care keeps his watch in every old man's eye,
And where care lodges, sleep will never lie."*

—SHAKESPEARE—

When we sleep, the body heals, the brain processes the new things we've learned and connects them with our life experience, and we awake well-rested, healthy, and ready to face the day's problems and frustrations. With so many well-known benefits, you're probably wondering: Why doesn't everyone make sleep a priority? Why doesn't my family listen when I tell them to sleep?

The problem is that restful sleep is not simply a matter of willpower or discipline.

If it were just a matter of good sleep hygiene, almost everyone would be getting good sleep. But sometimes, no matter what someone does, they can't get to sleep, stay asleep, or get the right kinds of sleep.

In this section of the book, I'm going to explain some of the ways that sleep goes wrong. We'll cover the things that keep people from getting a good night's sleep, even when they're trying. We'll look at how the brain falls apart without sleep and what that does to the rest of the body. Then, we'll look at the symptoms of sleep loss in children and adults because they don't always look the same. Finally, we'll dig into the long term consequences of sleep problems and why a lack of restful sleep may be the biggest health crisis facing America today.

I want to give you the facts and encouragement you need to spot sleep problems in your home, your extended family, and your community. Once you know what to look for, you'll be shocked at how many people you know aren't sleeping—and you'll be ready to know what you can do about it!

What Keeps Us Awake?

*"Care keeps his watch in every old man's eye,
And where care lodges, sleep will never lie."*

—William Shakespeare, Romeo and Juliet—

You try closing your eyes, but it doesn't do any good. Beside you, your spouse sleeps peacefully, blissfully unaware that you're lying there awake. *Curse them,* you think, resisting the urge to poke them until they join you on this slumberless night. You hear every noise in the house—the rattle of the window panes and the hum of the refrigerator torment you. You glance at the clock. Only six hours until morning. Tomorrow is going to be a terrible day.

You've been suffering from a bout of insomnia. Most people have occasional nights where they can't sleep, and they have a bad day or two and then recover. However, for some people, the bad sleep drags on for weeks, months, even years. We've talked about what scientists know about why and how people sleep, but what do we know about people who *don't* sleep? What does it mean when insomnia is permanent or when you think you're sleeping but wake up tired anyway?

Too Worried to Sleep

One of the reasons most people have trouble falling asleep or falling back asleep if they wake up is anxiety. For a person with anxiety, stressful thoughts make it impossible to fall asleep. Once they're asleep, they may wake in the night and be unable to get back to sleep. Then, the lack of sleep elevates the hormones that contribute to anxiety, and they can get stuck in a cycle of anxiety and sleep deprivation.

Scientists who study sleep have found that different kinds of anxiety affect sleep and sleep hormones in different ways. First of all, stress hormones from all kinds of anxiety promote a state of alertness and arousal since they're holding the body ready to fight or flee. This state is exactly the opposite of the relaxation needed to fall asleep and stay asleep all night.

It started after my mother died. Before, I'd always had a bedtime routine. A shower, a cup of cocoa, a book, and I'd be asleep in no time.

After her death, I started worrying. It wasn't depression, exactly. It was like being pelted with pebbles. All the things to do, all the things undone. Had I sent thank you notes for all the funeral flowers? Had I visited her grave enough? How was I going to clean out her house? How was I going to live without her voice on the phone or her hugs during the holidays?

As time went on, I lost the knack of falling asleep. Instead, I'd lay there, staring at the ceiling, worrying and making lists while the hours went by. I was achy, I was fuzzy, and I was sick all the time. My friends told me it was grief, that it would get better. But it was something more than grief. Other people with grief could sleep. I was lucky if I got two or three hours a night. I needed help and wasn't sure where to get it.

—Shana, age 34—

When a person is under social or psychological stress, it triggers a release of the corticotropin-releasing hormone. This hormone affects other hormonal systems, conscious behavior, and the autonomic system. It holds the whole body ready. While this hormone is sending signals to the brain, a person literally cannot relax.

In fact, there have been studies where this hormone is injected into healthy volunteers who do not have anxiety. If it is injected while a person is awake, they will be unable to fall asleep. Inject it into a sleeping person, and it either causes them to wake up frequently, or it reduces the amount of NREM sleep they get, affecting things like memory and hormonal balance.

For an anxious person, this creates a feedback loop, as hormones steal sleep, and lack of sleep causes more stress. Since we often treat sleep as a self-discipline issue, they face the added stigma of being told that willpower and good habits should result in sleep, even though the actual hormones controlling sleep are beyond their control.

There are also several specific mechanisms related to subtypes of anxiety:

Panic Attacks

Some people suffer from nighttime panic attacks. These attacks are most common in people whose daytime panic attacks happen when they can't be in a state of hyper-vigilance. These are the people who panic if things are too calm and quiet. Relaxing their guard gives them a feeling of impending disaster. Unfortunately, sleep also involves relaxing your guard and letting go. People with panic disorders may suffer multiple attacks a night and are often misdiagnosed. Over time, they may grow afraid of sleep.

General Anxiety Disorder (GAD)

People with GAD are usually able to fall asleep easily, but they can't *stay* asleep. They wake in the middle of the night and can't get back to sleep. With their sleep cut short, their GAD symptoms grow steadily worse.

Post Traumatic Stress Disorder (PTSD)

For PTSD patients, the main problem occurs during REM sleep. These patients have frequent, repetitive nightmares reliving their trauma. The nightmares are so unpleasant that these patients stop wanting to sleep, but without sleep, they can't process their fears or function during the day.

Obsessive-Compulsive Disorder (OCD)

Sleep lab studies done on patients with OCD have yielded an interesting result. Unlike other anxiety patients, this group doesn't sleep differently than a control group. Instead, they're just more prone to worry that their sleep isn't good enough, even though it's actually fine.

In the third part of the book, we'll address treatments for sleep disorders that help many patients, including anxiety patients. But for now, be aware that anxiety can steal sleep, and patients with diagnoses of anxiety should talk to their doctors about sleep issues and consider having a sleep study done to clarify what parts of sleep are affected by their illness.

Restless Legs, Restless Sleep

One common but under-diagnosed sleep issue is restless leg syndrome (RLS). RLS affects somewhere between ten to 24% of US adults and 2% of US children. It often worsens with age and can be linked to iron deficiencies, pregnancy, obesity, and sedentary jobs and lifestyles.

RLS can strike any time a person is still for a while, but it's especially bad in the evening and at night. People with RLS feel an unbearable urge to get up and move their legs. If they move around, they feel better for a while, but if they try to ignore it, it simply gets worse and worse until they can't focus on anything else.

RLS also comes with shame. A lot of adults and children who suffer from it have been berated or, in the case of children, punished for their inability to lie still without wiggling. But the disorder is based in the brain, and especially in how the brain reacts to dopamine.

Many people with RLS also suffer from Periodic Limb Movement of Sleep (PLMS). In PLMS, the patient's arms and legs twitch randomly, all night long, even during deep sleep. Sometimes, this can wake the sleeper, who then has to struggle with RLS in the attempt to sleep again. At other times, a spouse or roommate may complain about the constant twitching and thrashing all night. In both cases, the sleeper wakes less rested than they'd expect, given their bedtime and waking time.

In some people, there seems to be a connection between low ferritin levels and RLS. Ferritin is a measure of how much iron your body has stored. Many people with RLS have levels that are above the level for anemia but below average. For these people, treating the iron deficiency can improve or cure RLS.

Researchers are still not entirely sure why some people have RLS or why it gets worse with age. However, they're sure it's a neurological and sensory disorder, and the issue is somewhere in the brain. There is some evidence that people with RLS can benefit from vigorous exercise like running or swimming during the day.

NORMAL
CIRCADIAN RHYTHM   --- **NORMAL**

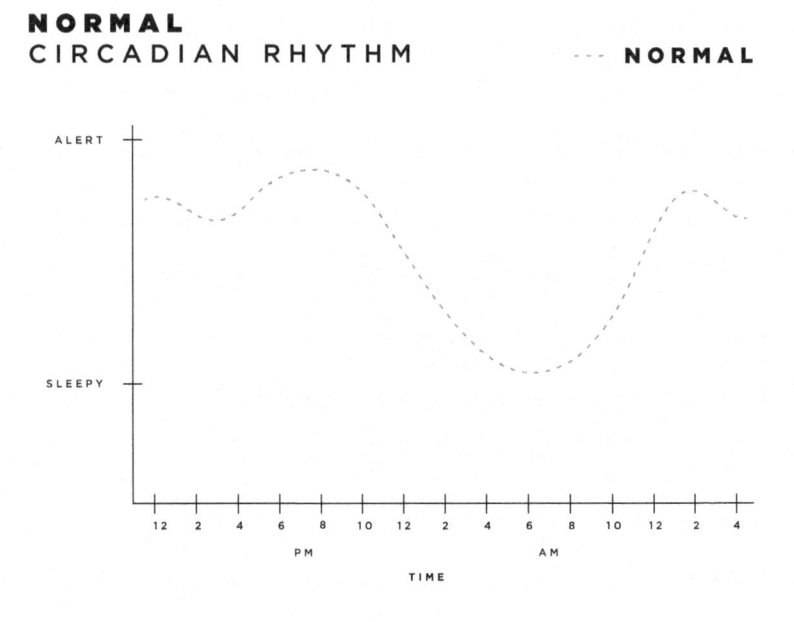

Figure 2. Here's a typical circadian rhythm. People grow more alert from the time they wake up until lunchtime. They typically experience a bout of sleepiness after lunch, and are then awake until their natural bedtime, when they grow very sleepy.

Out of Rhythm, Out of Sleep

Remember your circadian rhythms? They're the cycle that all living things have that tell you when to wake and when to sleep, when to eat and when to be active. Most people have circadian rhythms that roughly track to "normal" waking and sleep times, but some people are out of rhythm.

Your circadian rhythm is regulated by clock genes. Some people have mutations to these genes that shift them far off the schedule that society considers normal.

Extreme Night Owls

Keith was not a morning person, and it had become a running joke in the family. In college, he'd fail any class that started before 10:00 a.m. because he wouldn't manage to make it to tests and exams. When he worked in restaurants over the summers, the manager would have to call him to get him out of bed and into the kitchen. Luckily, he was a good worker once he got there, so he kept his job.

After he graduated, he kept keeping "student hours." He stayed up late, going out with friends or gaming, and had trouble pulling himself out of bed in the mornings. He had terrible performance reviews and drifted from job to job until he ended up working the second shift as an IT person. Suddenly, for the first time in his life, he was succeeding. Had he finally matured?

People with Delayed Sleep Phase Disorder (DSPD) naturally want to fall asleep between 1:00 a.m. and 6:00 a.m. and wake up between 9:00 a.m. and 2:00 p.m. These people have problems with morning classes or getting to work on time. If they do manage to wake up for an early class or shift, they'll often be sluggish and have difficulty learning until their brain wakes up. This disorder can be temporary, for instance, in teenagers, or it can be life-long.

NORMAL AND NIGHT OWL
CIRCADIAN RHYTHMS

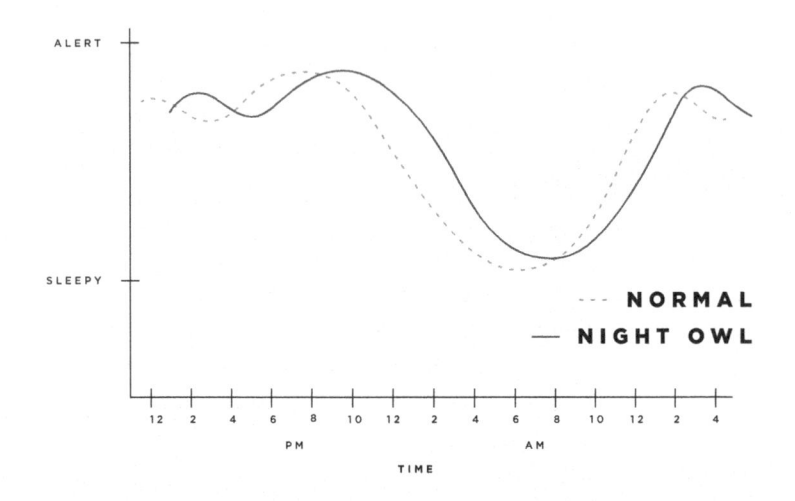

Figure 3. Night Owls fall asleep later and wake up later than a person with a normal cycle. DPSD is no joke. Many sufferers think they have insomnia, but they're really just out of phase with society's expectations.

Many people mistake DSPD for insomnia because they have trouble falling asleep. But the problem isn't actually insomnia; it's that their body clocks won't let them sleep during their natural "awake" time, any more than a healthy adult can fall asleep at 5:00 p.m.! Because the clock genes are hereditary, you may often see a strain of "extreme night owl" running in families. These are the people who are happiest and healthiest when they can work the second or third shift.

Because our society has a bias towards early risers, people with DSPD often have a lot of shame around their sleeping habits. They may have failed classes or lost jobs simply because they can't stay awake at certain times of the day. But about 10% of American adults fall into this group. A proper diagnosis can help them learn to work with their body's rhythms and find ways to optimize their life for their body's demands.

Up at the Crack of Dawn

On the flip side, some people's clock genes tell them to go to sleep as early as 6:00 p.m. and to wake up as early as 2:00 a.m. This is called Advanced Sleep Phase Disorder (ASPD). Sleep doctors aren't sure how common it is since the less severe cases want to sleep from 9:00 p.m. to 5:00 a.m. Since our society praises "early to bed and early to rise," many people with ASPD aren't even aware that they're outside the norm.

NORMAL AND EXTREME
MORNING CIRCADIAN RHYTHMS

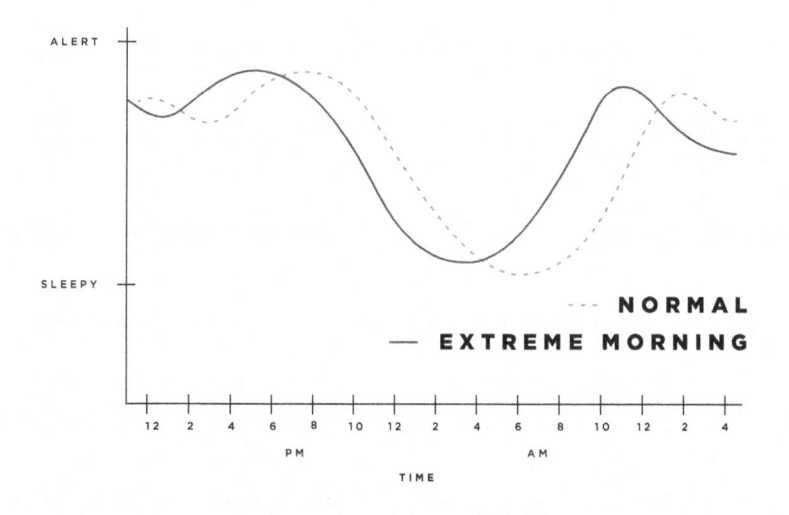

Figure 4. Early to bed and early to rise, gives you APSD, an extreme morning person. This can result in lost sleep, as it's not socially acceptable for a young person to go to bed at 7 and wake before dawn.

The problem comes when someone with the more severe sort forces themselves to stay awake until a "socially acceptable hour" that is three or four hours after their ideal bedtime. They may not have trouble falling asleep, but they're still awake at 2:00 or 3:00 a.m. Since they only got half a night's sleep, they'll be wide awake but also exhausted. They may find themselves relying on caffeine or other stimulants to make it through the day. Health effects add up because they can't balance the need for a nightlife and their need for sleep.

Why are rhythm disorders so common? Researchers think that it's because it's beneficial for society to have some people awake overnight and early in the morning. In the pre-industrial world, there were early morning farm chores, night watches against brigands, and the need to nurse people through the night. Today, factories, warehouses, hospitals, and emergency services all need people willing to work at odd hours. Many sleep disorders could improve if we just encouraged people to pick jobs whose schedules aligned with their natural rhythms.

Clocks Change with Age

Circadian rhythms also change with age. For instance, between ages twelve and about twenty-five, teens naturally switch to a later orientation. They want to stay up later and sleep later. How many of the mood swings and behavioral issues of the teen years are actually because we're forcing them to keep a child or adult schedule during this period of their life?

After middle age, many people start shifting to an earlier orientation. Many of the elderly find they're worn out by seven or eight at night and then wide awake in the early morning hours. There's a reason that "senior hour" at restaurants is often at 4:00 p.m. That's when seniors want their dinner! Again, many mood and mental effects of aging can be reduced if people just respect this change in their circadian rhythm.

Finally, in disorders such as Alzheimer's, the parts of the brain affecting the circadian rhythm can become unregulated. In some ways, it's almost like being a newborn again, untethered from the twenty-four-hour cycle of life. This leads to a fragmented sleep pattern, with naps at weird times, the "sundown effect" (which can look a lot like a colicky baby, but in a bigger, stronger person), and unpredictable hunger cues. The destruction of the brain's method for keeping us in rhythm shows us just how important knowing our circadian rhythms, and trying to live in accord with them, can be.

Melatonin Deficiencies

One new area of research is looking into whether deficiencies or processing issues with certain hormones can cause sleep disruptions and if there's a way to fix sleep in healthy ways with new kinds of medication. (Traditional sleep pills aren't actually healthy. They knock people out but don't let the brain do all the tasks of sleep.)

For instance, scientists are finding that many children on the autism spectrum have issues with how their bodies make and use melatonin. Remember how melatonin is the hormone that helps us get to sleep and stay asleep? Without it, or with too little of it, you may have a child who can't get to sleep or stay asleep. Up to 80% of kids with ASD have sleep issues, and the lack of sleep makes their symptoms worse. Some researchers think that the sleep issues early in development may even cause autism in some children. In the next few years, we may start seeing targeted intervention for the extreme sleep disruptions associated with autism so that kids and their parents can finally get a good night's rest.

The Take-Aways

- Anxiety can keep you from falling asleep and keep you awake if you get up between sleep cycles.

- Some sleep issues are actually vitamin and mineral deficiencies.

- Your circadian rhythms are controlled by your genes and are unchangeable. So your best bet is to work with them, not against them.

- Melatonin is important for sleep, and deficiencies in it can cause all sorts of problems.

Try This

The next time you have a week off of work, take a sleep vacation. No plans, no alarms, just you and your circadian rhythms. See when you get up and when you get sleepy when you don't need to adjust your clock to the world's.

Things to Think About

- Who in your extended family is a night owl? Who is a morning person? Can you see any patterns?

- Can you rearrange your life to better fit your rhythms?

- Is anxiety keeping you awake? What tools can you use to wind down for bed?

- Do you have RLS or other sleep issues? When was the last time you had routine bloodwork done?

4

Stolen Breath, Stolen Sleep

"Hark, how hard he fetches breath."

WILLIAM SHAKESPEARE, KING HENRY IV, PART 1—

As you saw in the last chapter, there are many reasons why people can't get to sleep and stay asleep. But what if you put yourself to bed at the same time every night, wake up in the morning, and are still tired and draggy all day long? What could be going on?

> *It happened so gradually I didn't even notice. I took good care of myself. I exercised, ate my vegetables, made sure to go to bed on time. Yet somehow, my health markers were all moving in the wrong direction. My weight was going up, my blood pressure*

was nuts, and I was pre-diabetic on a healthy diet. It was like there was no longer any connection between my behavior and my body. I was in bed nine and a half or ten hours a day, so why did I feel so awful?

—MELISSA, AGE 45—

Your brain and body need sleep to repair, to grow, to optimize themselves for your life. But to do the work of sleep, your body needs oxygen. Our lungs take in air, remove the oxygen, and transport it to every cell in the body. Oxygen is essential for cellular respiration, the act of extracting energy from sugar to fuel our bodies. Without enough oxygen, your cells can't use glucose to make energy. And without energy, your body can't do its work.

Have you ever been short of breath during the day? Have you ever had smoke from a bonfire catch you in the face? Have you had pneumonia or bronchitis? Do you have asthma? If you've had to struggle to breathe, you know how scary it can be. You gasp and choke, your lungs ache. It's a struggle to stand up or walk or think. Your body can't function without oxygen. You feel like you're going to die.

Many people have this exact same sensation when they're sleeping. But since they're asleep while they're struggling to breathe, they don't remember it in the morning. They wake up feeling tired, like they've fought a battle all night, but they don't know why. But even if they don't remember the time they've spent without enough oxygen, their body remembers. The work of sleep is left undone. They may even be in worse shape than they were before they went to bed. As days and weeks and months drag on, the lack of oxygen at night takes a larger and larger toll until they finally notice and get help.

This condition of not being able to get enough oxygen at night is called ***Sleep Disordered Breathing (SDB)***. For people with SDB, sleep is no longer restorative. It's being stolen away. And since many people with SDB breathe fine during the day and embrace healthy lifestyles, they may not even notice the damage that's slowly occurring throughout their bodies.

There are many causes of sleep-disordered breathing, and if you suspect that you or someone you love is suffering from it, you need an evaluation. I'd like to go over a few of the most common causes of SDB so that you can understand why you are struggling at night and why it's not your fault or a reason for shame.

Allergic Rhinitis

"Everyone has seasonal allergies," I told myself. "It's no big deal. I can just soldier through." My wife complained about my snoring, but I figured she was just being melodramatic. Sure, I was draggy and cranky, but it would be better after we had a hard freeze, so why was everyone complaining?

She insisted on coming to my next appointment, and she showed the doctor a recording she'd made of my snoring. I wasn't just making noise. I was literally gagging and gasping for breath. All this time, I'd been blaming being tired on allergies, but it turned out that it was how I slept that was hurting me.

—Allan, Age 47—

About one-third of adults suffer from allergic rhinitis. When they're around things like pollen, dust, mold, or animal dander, their noses get stuffy, their sinuses swell shut, and drainage pours down the back of their throats. This can have a huge impact on the quality of their sleep.

For many people with allergies, bedrooms are a hotspot. Dust is a common allergen. Where does it come from? Dust mites are tiny creatures that have evolved to live near humans, eating our dead skin. This is a good thing—who wants piles of dead skin everywhere? The problem is these tiny creatures—they're microscopic—don't just eat. They also poop and die, leaving tiny pieces of their bodies everywhere.

This rubbish is stirred up by air currents, and we inhale it. When someone who is allergic to dust mites inhales little bits of dust mite bodies, it triggers an allergic reaction. Their body attacks the particles as if they were a virus or bacteria. And so, they get symptoms similar to those that you get with a common cold.

Where do you find more dust mites? Wherever there's more dead skin. They love living on dirty laundry, in carpets and drapes, and especially in your bedding. That means that at night, as you sleep, you're inhaling dust. For many people with allergies, everything spins out of control at night.

Normally, people breathe through their noses. This ensures that the lungs get air that's been appropriately filtered and humidified by the nose and sinuses. But during an allergy attack, those pathways are no longer clear. Either the sleeper struggles to breathe through the narrowed sinuses, or they start mouth breathing. This leads to snoring, dry air that irritates the breathing passages, choking and gagging on phlegm, and ultimately a drop in oxygen levels and gasping.

Because this often happens in deep-sleep, the sleeper isn't aware of what's going on. They may not even realize they have nighttime allergy attacks if dust is their main allergen.

Dust mites are stealing their sleep and damaging their health. Unless they have a housemate who complains about the snoring and coughing, they may not know until it's too late to reverse the damage.

If you wake up stuffy in the mornings or with a sore throat, get screened for sleep breathing issues. Allergic rhinitis seems minor, but if it's left untreated, it can spiral into other, worse issues with your sleep breathing.

Asthma

Before we got treatment, she'd cough on and off all night. I could barely sleep myself! I'd just lie awake, listening. "Cough cough cough, cough cough cough." Then she'd stop, and I'd catch my breath, wondering if she'd died or just had a moment of normal breathing. And then it would start again, on and off, a couple of times a week, all through the year.

During the day, she was fine. She was the fasted runner on her soccer team and never had to stop and catch her breath. She didn't wheeze. She didn't have obvious allergies like peanuts or shellfish. It was just the coughing at night. Until I happened to mention it at a checkup, I didn't realize what a big deal it was. I thought it was just something I had to live with, the coughing and the worrying.

—MOTHER OF CHEYENNE, AGE 8—

If allergies are bad for sleep breathing, asthma is even worse. About 8% of the US population suffers from some form of asthma, and it's often worse for children than adults because their airways are narrower. For many asthmatics, nighttime is a dangerous time.

According to the Sleep Foundation, this is because everyone's airway function decreases the longer that they sleep. In a healthy person, this doesn't really matter—even decreased function means adequate oxygen. However, for an asthmatic, any decrease can cause serious breathing issues.

The breathing passages of an asthmatic child or adult respond to certain triggers by both becoming inflamed and swelling and by narrowing. The combination means that it can be hard to get any air at all, so they begin coughing and wheezing. For some asthmatics, this mostly happens at night, so they may sleep through the coughing fits and not realize that their brain spent the night starved for oxygen.

Asthma triggers vary a lot from person to person. They may be related to allergies, but attacks can also be caused by acid reflux, changes in the weather, emotional stress, or infection. Over time, untreated or undertreated asthma can cause permanent damage to the respiratory system.

A nagging nighttime cough is a sign that someone isn't breathing well in their sleep, even if they don't fully wake up as they cough. It interrupts the work of sleep and leaves brains and bodies unready for the new day.

When the Brain Can't Find the Rhythm

Sometimes, a problem in the brain can cause sleep-disordered breathing. For instance, premature babies sometimes experience Apnea of Prematurity. Their brains aren't developed enough to breathe in a regular rhythm, and they can stop breathing until a nurse rubs their back and reminds them to breathe again. Eventually, the baby's brain matures enough so that they can breathe consistently, day and night.

When an adult's brain can't maintain regular breathing during sleep, it's known as central sleep apnea (CSA). CSA is relatively rare. While some people seem hard-wired not to breathe, most people with CSA develop it as a result of illness, injury, or medication.

Patients with heart failure can suffer from CSA because their heart is unable to pump blood throughout the body. As a result, they can alternate between hyperventilating and extremely slow and sometimes stopped breathing in an effort to better control the oxygen level in the blood. Stroke victims may also have CSA. In both cases, patients may need oxygen tanks to help their breathing become more efficient at transferring oxygen to the blood.

Atrial fibrillation and narcotics use can also cause CSA. In all of these cases, you might notice a family member breathing very quickly and then not breathing at all. They may not snore or gasp. CSA is a serious condition and should be assessed by a medical professional as soon as possible.

Obstructive Sleep Apnea

I live alone, so I had no idea anything was wrong with me. But I was tired and depressed. My blood pressure was through the roof, and no matter how much I exercised, I kept gaining weight. I was fuzzy-brained too. I used to have a great memory; I hardly needed a calendar to remember appointments and deadlines. Now, I had to write everything down, and sometimes even that didn't help.

I chalked it up to getting older. I mean, I was in my 50s, and maybe this was just the beginning of a long, slow decline. An off-hand comment to my doctor about my morning headaches triggered a screening and evaluation. So much of what I'd thought was an unavoidable part of aging was bad sleep-breathing! I haven't felt this good in a decade, and I'm so thankful my doctor was on the ball.

—Joe, age 53—

One of the most common and under-treated forms of SDB is obstructive sleep apnea (OSA). In OSA, the brain is sending the proper signals, the lungs can oxygenate the blood, but physical features are blocking the flow of air during sleep. For someone with OSA, sleep is not restful or restorative.

Instead, the sleeper struggles to get air through a narrowed or totally blocked airway. They snort, snore, and grunt. Periodically, they stop breathing altogether then gasp for air. If you hook a patient with OSA up to sleep-tracking equipment, you get a disturbing look into how airway issues are stealing their sleep and their lives.

A person with OSA can't achieve deeper stages of NREM sleep for very long. Instead, every time they stop breathing, their blood oxygen level plummets. This, in turn, puts the brain into a panic. Stress hormones course through their veins, their heart rate rockets, they wake up for a second or two, gasp for air, and then fall back asleep.

In the morning, the sleeper won't remember these microarousals. However, the frequent, tiny awakenings mean that their body doesn't rest, the restorative work of NREM doesn't occur, and their memories and ability to learn new things are injured. Over time, months and years of sleep apnea ruin their bodies, wreck their minds, and shorten their lives.

OSA affects children and adults, men and women. While there's a stereotype that only obese people suffer from OSA, many young, thin people also struggle with it. Because diagnosis requires a night in a sleep lab, many people are unaware that they have this disease and that when they sleep, instead of healing, their body is undergoing massive harm as it weathers frequent oxygen loss and huge stress to the system.

What exactly is Apnea?

An apnea event is when breathing totally stops because of the blocked airway. No air is getting through. A hypopnea event is when the airway is partially blocked. In a healthy adult, your blood oxygen saturation should stay above 95% all night. When it drops below 92%, that's a sign of apnea or hypopnea and means your brain isn't getting enough sleep.

Even a healthy adult may have some low oxygen events in a night. In OSA, the sleeper experiences more than five of these microarousals every hour. That's enough to disrupt the work of sleep and create lasting mental and physical damage.

How do they measure the severity of Apneas?

When your airway is blocked, and you can only get 20-50% of your normal airflow, that's called a **hypopnea**. If your airflow drops below 20%, that's an **apnea**. Sleep scientists combine these two pieces of data into the Apnea-Hypopnea Index (AHI). Your **AHI** is the average number of apneas and hypopneas you experience in an hour. For an adult, an AHI greater than or equal to five means that you are having a problem with sleep breathing. In a child, even an AHI of one is enough for a diagnosis of OSA.

Many insurers use the AHI to determine what sorts of treatments they'll cover. Unfortunately, using AHI alone misses about 30% of people who have sleep breathing problems. That's the 30% of patients who are in the earlier stages of SDB and whose condition will progress, causing life-altering damage if it's not treated.

The American Academy of Sleep Medicine (AASM) prefers to use a different, more precise tool called the Respiratory Disturbance Index (**RDI**). The RDI differs from the AHI because it also includes **RERA**s. A RERA is a respiratory event-related arousal. These are those microarousals that cause so many problems, especially during deep sleep. When someone wakes up for a few seconds to move so that they can breathe better, that is included in the RDI.

This is important because many people will struggle to breathe or wake and change position before their difficulty rises to the level of apnea or hypopnea. The work of sleep is disrupted in these people just as if they'd completely stopped breathing for a moment. And, as time goes on, someone with many RERAs will gain weight or suffer cardiovascular damage, and their condition will progress until they finally have full-blown apneas.

What is Obstructing the Airway?

In OSA, the airway is physically blocked. While someone with allergies or asthma may have inflammation narrowing their airways, in OSA, it's structural. That means that medication like steroids or albuterol can't relieve the blockage. OSA is a blanket term for many different physical issues, and the issues causing OSA can vary with age, other health conditions, and genetics.

TONSILS
AND **THROAT**

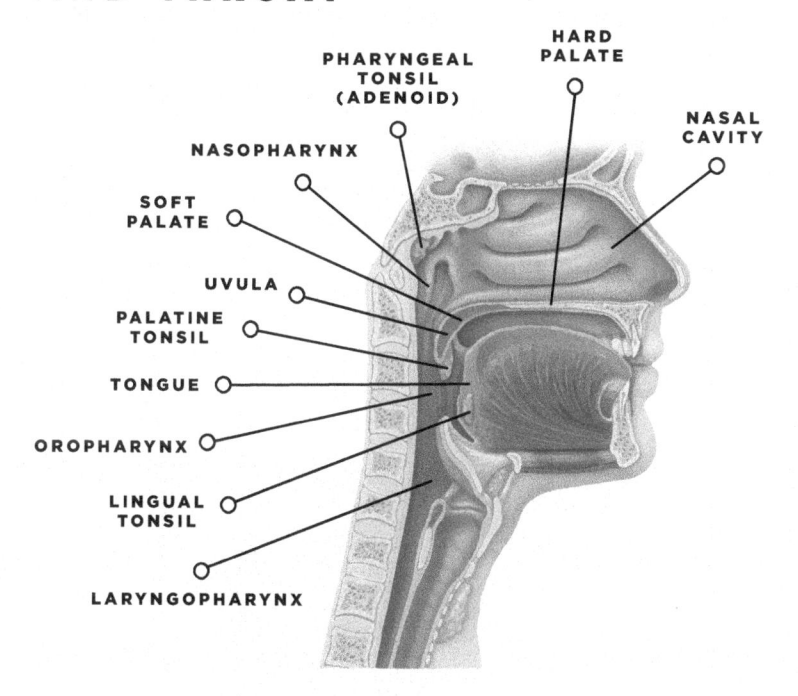

Labels on diagram: PHARYNGEAL TONSIL (ADENOID), HARD PALATE, NASAL CAVITY, NASOPHARYNX, SOFT PALATE, UVULA, PALATINE TONSIL, TONGUE, OROPHARYNX, LINGUAL TONSIL, LARYNGOPHARYNX

Figure 5. Your upper airways are complicated, and have many different parts. When any part of the airway is enlarged, mispositioned, blocked, or not working correctly, it can cause big problems for your sleep breathing.

Enlarged Tonsils and Adenoids

For many children with OSA, the blockage is caused by enlarged tonsils and adenoids. Tonsils and adenoids are glands in the throat that are part of the immune system. When you inhale a virus or bacteria, the tonsils and adenoids can stop it, release antibodies, and prevent the disease from reaching your lungs. Adenoids also move mucus from the sinuses into the stomach to prevent infectious agents from reaching the lungs.

When tonsils and adenoids are involved in fighting a disease like mono or flu, they can swell up. This is why so many viruses cause a sore throat or swollen neck. Tonsils and adenoids are most active in fighting infection from birth until age seven. Then they start shrinking. In most healthy adults, they are tiny and rarely swollen at all.

T&A DIAGRAM FOR SURGERY

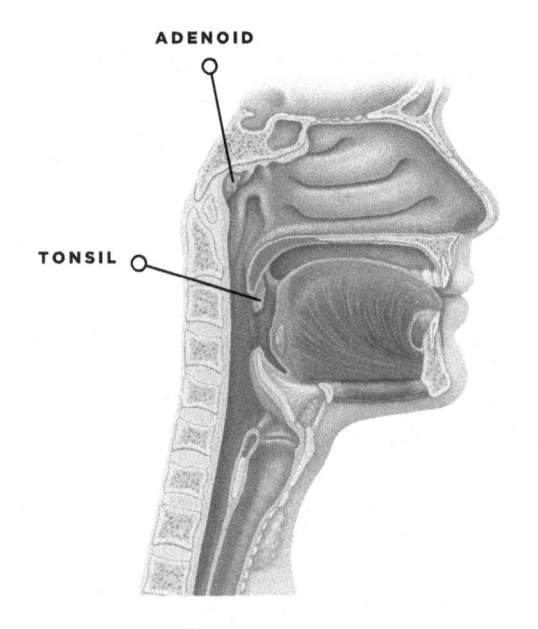

Figure 6. In a small child, enlarged tonsils and adenoids can combine with a narrower airway to cause big sleep breathing problems.

In some kids, they're extra-large compared to the size of the airway. Or, if a child has a chronic strep infection or is a mouth breather, they may become permanently irritated and swollen. In some children, the tonsils are so enlarged they practically touch. During sleep, hyper-enlarged tonsils and adenoids can block off the airway, causing apnea. If the problem is severe enough, immune problems caused by a lack of healthy sleep can outweigh the immune benefits that the tonsils and adenoids provide.

Maria, small for her age and slow at school, was always sitting around slack-jawed, her mouth partially open. Her parents and teachers would tell her to close her mouth and sit up straight, but as soon as the adults weren't looking, her mouth would open again. The mouth breathing was causing problems with bad breath and tooth pain, so Maria's parents brought her to a pediatric dentist.

After a screening, the dentist did an examination. Just as she'd suspected, Maria had "kissing tonsils." She suspected the adenoids were also swollen. Maria was a mouth breather because she couldn't get air any other way, and the same habit that was affecting her appearance during the day was impacting her breathing at night. Maria's parents left the office with a referral to a pediatric ear, nose, and throat specialist. Their daughter was finally going to get the help she needed to breathe, sleep, learn, and grow.

Big Neck

For adults, the size of the neck can contribute to sleep apnea. If your neck is larger than normal (greater than seventeen inches around for men or sixteen inches around for women), it can mean that fat is surrounding your airway. This fat can tighten the opening, making it harder to breathe and causing snoring and hypopneas in the night.

Even worse, if you sleep on your back, the weight of your neck can collapse the airway or change the position of the tongue and completely block it. Many people with sleep apnea often end up sleeping on their sides because it helps keep the weight of their necks off their airways.

High Palate

One structural issue that can cause sleep apnea is a high, arched palate. Nasal breathing is healthy breathing, especially during sleep. When someone has a very high, arched palate, it changes the shape of their sinuses and blocks the flow of air. For someone with a high palate, even a small amount of inflammation or mucus can block the sinuses.

NARROW PALATE **NORMAL PALATE**

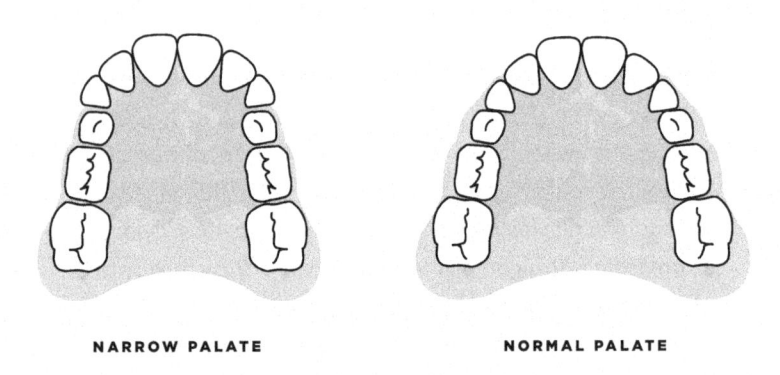

Figure 7. With a narrow palate, also known as a Gothic arch, the teeth are crowded and the roof of the mouth is smaller. In a normal palate, also called a Roman arch, there is plenty of room for the teeth and the broad roof of the mouth means that the nasal cavity is larger.

How does a sleeper respond when the nasal passages and sinuses are blocked? They open their mouth and try to take in air that way. Mouth breathing can cause several problems. The tongue is more likely to get in the way of the airflow, reducing oxygen. The air that does enter the windpipe is going to be colder and drier and cause the tonsils, adenoids, and throat to swell while irritating the lungs. With a high palate, you'll get more snoring, more mouth breathing, and more irritation. All of this leads to more effort to breathe and lower blood oxygen during sleep.

Tongue-Tie

Tongue-tie works with the high palate to further complicate night breathing. A tied, or tethered, tongue can't move freely around the mouth. An untethered tongue can rest on the roof of the mouth during sleep. During childhood, your tongue naturally expands and flattens your palate to make room for adult teeth and to give you wider nasal passages. If the tongue is tied, it can't rest on the roof. Instead, it will flop backward in the throat, blocking the airway and dropping oxygen levels during sleep.

TONGUE TIE HIGH PALATE CUTAWAY DIAGRAM

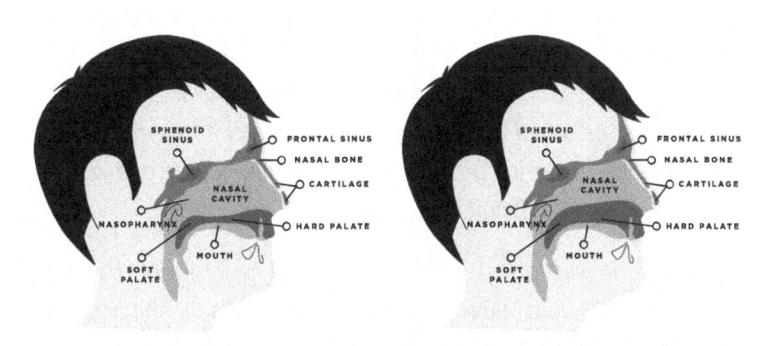

Figure 8. In a normal child (left) the nasal cavity has a broad, flat base that allows for easy breathing. In a child with tongue tie (right), a high, narrow palate obstructs the free flow of air through the nasal cavity.

In the past, tongue tie wasn't a large cause of sleep apnea in children and young adults because most pediatricians clipped the tissue tethering it at birth. However, in recent years doctors don't routinely clip tongue ties. If a baby has feeding issues and starts losing weight, they'll intervene. Otherwise, they leave the tongue as it is. The problem is that a tongue tie may be mild enough to allow weight gain yet still severe enough to cause sleep apnea.

Jack's mom knew that his tongue didn't seem to work as other kids' did. He'd always been prone to gagging and choking when he ate. Food seemed to get stuck in his cheeks, and he never quite knew how to chew and swallow well. She just assumed it was sensory issues or something and never thought to bring it up with his pediatrician.

He was a hard child all around. As a baby, he'd nursed round the clock and screamed if she tried to put him down. He was hyperactive, a tightly wound ball of destructive energy. His emotions were up and down. He'd burst into tears without warning, and it seemed like other kids delighted in pushing his buttons to make him angry. He never seemed to sleep. He'd go down at bedtime, only to bounce out of bed a few hours later. He was an only child, and his mother never sought an evaluation. She just assumed he was high strung and a bit immature. She tried one parenting program after another, hoping one would work with her difficult child.

When he was in first grade, he also had major problems with reading. He didn't have his l's or r's, and as a result, phonics was a major struggle. He was on the waitlist for a speech therapist evaluation. Around this time, the family's insurance changed, and they switched dentists. During the first exam, the doctor turned to his mother and asked, "Did anyone ever tell you that your son has a severe tongue-tie? It's probably affecting his speech, his eating, and his sleep."

Fatty Tongue

When people gain weight, they don't just gain fat in the parts of the body we can see. They also gain fat internally. Researchers are discovering that for many people with obesity, tongue fat plays a major role in OSA. Fat slightly constricts the airway while increasing the size of the tongue.

When the tongue has gotten fatty, it can block the windpipe when it relaxes during sleep. Air from the nose can't get past it easily. As the air is forced through the narrow opening, it makes the familiar snoring noise. In extreme cases, the fat on the tongue may completely block the airway when someone lies on their back.

Scientists have also discovered that some people can have abnormal fat deposits on their tongue even when they themselves are a healthy weight. This can cause all the same issues with sleep breathing, but they may miss out on screening and diagnosis because so many doctors only look for OSA in obese patients.

Soft Palate Collapse

Take your tongue, and press it against the roof of your mouth near your teeth. Do you feel how hard that is? That's your hard palate. Now, without breaking contact, move it backward. Can you feel where your hard palate ends and your soft palate begins?

Your soft palate is a combination of muscle and tissue that helps keep food and liquid out of your respiratory system. When you swallow, it blocks off the entrance to your nose. When you're eating, it lets you breathe and chew at the same time.

With age, your soft palate can lose some of its muscle tone and get floppy. Then, at night, it can collapse and block your airway while you're sleeping, contributing to OSA. Some researchers have suggested that years of snoring can contribute to this collapse, as the constant vibrations can weaken the muscle and other tissue.

Epiglottis collapse

In rare cases, OSA can be caused by epiglottis collapse instead of soft palate collapse. Then the epiglottis, which usually protects the windpipe during swallowing, blocks it during sleep. This most often happens in people who've had head or neck surgeries, certain kinds of strokes, or chemotherapy for the head and neck. Because of the direction of the collapse, traditional OSA interventions will actually make the condition worse in people with epiglottic collapse.

UARS: Overlooked and Underdiagnosed

If you're middle-aged, overweight, and have other conditions like high blood pressure, most medical practitioners will suggest that breathing issues are robbing you of some of your sleep. But there's another form of SDB that affects your ability to rest well. Your blood oxygen may never drop very low, but that's because you're waking yourself up to respond to breathing troubles. In this case, you have many microarousals, but your other symptoms may not look like sleep disordered-breathing…yet.

Upper Airway Resistance Syndrome, or UARS, is a syndrome where it's difficult to breathe during sleep because air can't move freely through your upper airways. This can be caused by many different issues, including:

- deformities in the nose and sinuses
- chronic infections
- polyps
- swelling from allergies
- muscle problems
- the shape of your palate
- an overbite that affects jaw position and airway shape during sleep

Often, people with UARS are loud snorers. They don't stop breathing during sleep, but their bad breathing causes them to frequently toss and turn, wake up to move pillows, or readjust their head and neck during sleep. They won't remember doing these things, but they all interrupt the work of sleep.

People suffering from UARS may report being tired or run-down, but they often don't appear sick enough to trigger an OSA screen. The problem is that they're racking up years of bad sleep. Over time, the struggles to breathe and the vibrations from snoring can cause damage to the soft palate, neck muscles, and carotid arteries. Ignored, UARS becomes OSA, and damage becomes irreversible.

What does this mean for my family and me?

When you suspect a loved one has SDB, it's important to learn about underlying causes. The source of breathing issues will matter for the treatment and long-term outcomes. In the next chapter, you'll learn how lack of sleep from SDB or other causes affects the brain, both in the short and the long-term, and why it's not OK to put off screening and treatment.

The Take-Aways

- Allergies and asthma can impact sleep in a big way. Make sure that your family's bedrooms make good breathing a priority.

- Snoring is a sign that something is wrong with your sleep breathing.

- Mild sleep-disordered breathing (SDB) will often progress to full-blown obstructive sleep apnea (OSA) if left untreated.

- UARS and OSA are both very common in the US.

Try This

Do you snore? Ask your family. Does anyone in your family snore? If the answer is yes, make a doctor's appointment ASAP.

Things to Think About

- Who in your family snores? Coughs at night? Wakes up with a dry mouth? Gets morning headaches? Are they being treated for sleep breathing issues?
- If not, what's keeping you from bringing up these issues with your medical team? Can you contact them?
- If you woke up truly refreshed and reinvigorated each day, how would that change your life?

5

The Sleepless Brain

"I've always envied people who sleep easily. Their brains must be cleaner, the floorboards of the skull well swept, all the little monsters closed up in a steamer trunk at the foot of the bed."

—David Benioff, *City of Thieves*—

One of the biggest problems with sleep is that we need *all* of it to function well. The light and deep NREM sleep, unbroken for long stretches, the REM that gets more frequent as daybreak approaches, the hour after hour of repeated sleep cycles—you need all of these to be able to function. And since the brain controls so much of our conscious and unconscious behavior, when it can't do the work of sleep, things start going haywire.

Earlier in this book, I talked about what sleep does for the brain and body and why we need it. In this chapter, I'm going to give you more specifics of what happens to you in the short term when you aren't getting enough good sleep.

It started with a prescription for beta blockers for a stubborn blood pressure issue. Elena wasn't thrilled with the initial dizziness and exhaustion, but as time went on, she got used to it. Blood pressure issues were dangerous, so she'd stay on the pills even though she was a little fuzzier and a little draggier. After about a month, she could drive again, and she just kept pushing through the symptoms.

"They'd told me sleep disruption was a rare side effect," she explains, "so I didn't look for it."

Her husband and kids noticed first. "Are you going senile?" Elena's teen daughter demanded. She regularly had no memory of things that her husband and children said had happened in the last few days or weeks. There was just a haze where memories should be.

She started getting more and more tired. She was sick all the time. Where once, she could hike five or eight miles without getting tired, now she couldn't load or unload the dishwasher without frequent breaks. Elena was spending sixteen to eighteen hours a day in bed but couldn't figure out why. Her blood pressure was still pretty high, she was taking more and more of the medicines, and she just kept feeling worse and worse.

Before, she'd frequently had vivid, memorable dreams. Now it seemed like she didn't dream at all. She was just so tired. But somehow, she couldn't figure out why.

She was at the doctor for a check-up when she broke down crying and explained the struggle of the last few months and how her life was falling apart. He stopped the beta-blockers that day. Within a month, she had her old self back. And she remembered her dreams again.

One problem with stolen sleep is that it affects the brain. And the brain is exactly the part of your body you need to recognize the patterns that show you're not sleeping. In my practice, it's often a parent or spouse who brings in someone for screening. The patient has no idea anything is wrong because their brain is too exhausted to notice all the signs of sleep deprivation. Learning, memories, mental health, and personality all change when a person cannot sleep.

Learning and the Sleepless Brain

Think about the times in your life you've had to study hard for something, like a test in school, a certification exam, or even a driver's test. You studied hard but might have felt like you didn't really get it. Then, on the day of the test, much to your surprise, you passed! The work the brain does during sleep helped change your studying into usable knowledge.

So, what happens when people are trying to learn new things, but they're not getting enough high quality sleep to let the brain do its work? As you might expect, nothing good.

Remember how sleep clears out the hypothalamus so that you can learn new things? When someone isn't getting enough sleep, they can't clear out their short term memory all the way. They have less room to learn new things. This is one reason small children need naps. Learning language takes a huge effort, and napping one or two times a day lets them keep learning.

For adults, the same thing happens. Most of us learn more quickly in the morning than in the evening. The things that we try to learn right before bed are less likely to "stick" than the material that we learned earlier in the day because our brain is full. They're trying to learn at the time of day when their brain is least able to handle new things.

If you cut back on sleep or pull all-nighters, you learn even less. And over the long-term, lack of sleep can have huge effects on learning. College students who are sleep deprived in the month, or even the week, before a test score much lower than students who prioritize sleep.

In fact, experts think as much as 25% of the difference in students' class performance is because of sleep. That means that if you have a child or teen who isn't sleeping well, they're struggling in school. They're working harder for less reward than their peers whose brains have time to do the work of sleep.

Language and motor skills are especially dependent on slow-wave sleep. During this time, the brain transfers memories and rehearses the new skills. For language learners, REM is also important since it helps them build connections with what they already know.

So, if you're an adult who doesn't sleep, what do you think happens when there's a new computer program at work, you get a new car with controls in slightly different places, or even if your favorite social media site changes its user interface yet again?

Just like a school kid or college student, you have trouble learning. You can't do as well at your job because you can't learn from new experiences at work. You're not as good a driver because you can't learn new routes or new vehicles quickly and well. You're slow using new technology and want to yell at your phone. You feel foggy and confused because everything is changing, and your brain can't keep up with it. You've lost the neuroplasticity you need to learn because you're not sleeping.

One final way sleep loss affects learning is because of a part of the brain called the myelin sheath. Myelin is a fatty layer that helps keep signals from getting weaker as the brain sends them back and forth—think of it as the insulation on a wire. Children get more myelin as they grow, and this myelinization happens while they sleep. Adults repair myelin during sleep.

When myelin can't be made or repaired, signals get weaker or lost. Your working memory is smaller and slower. It's difficult to do things like read or solve equations. In fact, myelinization seems to play a role in things like phonics and math learning, and kids who don't have enough are more likely to have learning disabilities.

When a child, or even an adult, isn't getting enough sleep, defects in the myelin layer can make learning and problem-solving a lot harder. Your brain feels fried after a few nights of bad sleep because it's no longer able to transmit signals efficiently. And for a kid with undiagnosed sleep issues, who may never have had the chance to lay down a good layer of myelin? Their brain is "fried" all the time. Lack of sleep is making it much harder to learn. Every night that they can't do the work of sleep, they fall farther and farther behind their classmates.

When Sleep is Just a Memory, Memories Aren't

We're made of memories—it's why stories about people with amnesia are so fascinating. A night, or a year of nights, of bad sleep won't give you amnesia, but sleep loss does chip away at your memory. Over time, you may find yourself growing fuzzier, slower, and less competent. You might blame it on stress or aging, but the problem is a lot more basic—and more solvable.

Well, I Declare...

Quick, what was your fourth-grade teacher's name? What was the address of your childhood home? What color was your grandma's bathtub? These sound like quiz questions for a forgotten password, but they're also examples of declarative memory. Declarative memory is your ability to recall and communicate facts like the names of old neighbors or the answers to a history test.

Sleep is essential for both making new declarative memories and accessing old ones. When you haven't slept or haven't slept well, you have trouble finding these names, words, or dates. It's on the tip of your tongue; you feel yourself reaching for it but can't grab it. You *know* the words, but you just can't think them or say them.

These feelings are an accurate description of what's going on in a sleep-deprived brain. It's not that your stored memories have been erased—you remembered that Mrs. Grandview lived next door yesterday, and you'll remember it tomorrow if you sleep. The memory is still there. Lack of sleep has destroyed the pathways you use to access these memories.

In fact, people are beginning to suspect that much of the mental fuzziness associated with perimenopause and menopause in women may be a result of disturbed sleep. So, when you ask your child to get "the thing that I left in that room" because you can't remember words, it may be a sign that it's time to get screened for sleep issues.

And in Our Next Episode...

Declarative memories are for facts, but sleep also affects your episodic memory. Episodic memory is what most people talk about when they say "memories." They include all five senses and emotions about events from your past.

Think about walking into your grandmother's kitchen while she cooked, getting ready to give a speech in front of your class, or standing at the graveside for a beloved uncle's burial. These are strong memories that make you who you are. When you call them up, either deliberately or because some smell or feel in the air reminded you of them, it's like you're in the moment. You remember how you felt, how things smelled, why you cared.

When you're not getting enough sleep, your existing episodic memories are fine. What sleep deprivation changed is your ability to make *new* episodic memories. Someone who's not sleeping enough will lack strong episodic memories from the periods of sleep deprivation.

Think back to a time with a newborn or when you were working a hard job. When you ask people about those times, they'll often say, "It's all kind of a blur." That blur is the lack of good episodic memory. Without those memories, your connection to the past is dulled. You miss out on strong emotional memories. It's harder to connect with the people who shared those moments with you.

Since episodic memory represents how we've learned and grown, when we lose it, we lose something of ourselves. One reason older people often have crystal clear memories of youth and very fuzzy ones of recent events is that their sleep is shorter and less efficient. Memory loss is partially a loss of the ability to make *new* memories, and sleep plays a role.

If you're not sleeping well, you won't notice that you're not making clear memories of your current life—until someone else asks you about a shared event, and you realize you literally cannot remember it at all.

Now, Where Was I?

How do you deal with interruptions? If you, or someone you love, is sleep-deprived, the answer is probably "very poorly." If a sleep-deprived person is completing a list of steps like a recipe, a surgical routine, or a chore list, interruptions can derail the whole process.

Sleep interferes with your working memory, that is, the ability to hold the facts you're using right now where you can use them. A sleep-deprived waitress will forget your order on the way to the kitchen unless she writes it down. A sleep-deprived child may wander off while getting dressed for school, one sock on and one sock off. Without working memory, interruptions mean forgetting everything.

This has terrible effects on our society. If you're sleep-deprived and baking and accidentally add the salt twice, it's no big deal. But if you're a surgeon, you might leave a sponge inside a patient and sew them back up, or forget to wash your hands well before examining someone. If you're a truck driver, you might forget to check your mirror before changing lanes. If you're a kid at school, you might forget instructions and get punished for being bad or defiant when you really can't remember at all.

Life is full of interruptions, so when your working memory doesn't work, you don't work. If you don't get enough sleep, you'll make more mistakes, stop working more, and forget what you're doing. As the months go by, you'll start to get a reputation as someone who is fuzzy and ditzy. You might blame the change on aging or stress, but the root cause is lack of sleep. Until you fix your sleep, you won't be able to fix your working memory.

Two Left Feet

Earlier, I told you about the important role sleep plays in learning new motor skills. Typing, writing, driving, dancing, sports—to improve these skills, you need sleep. So what happens when you deprive people of sleep, so they only get six or seven hours for months on end?

Sleep-deprived people are clumsier. When a rat is deprived of sleep, he has trouble learning to navigate a new maze. When a person is sleep-deprived, they may spend a week bumping into that file cabinet that just got moved. Their brain can't catch up with the sequence needed to move through a new space, and it looks like clumsiness.

Sleep-deprived athletes get injured more. They aren't learning as much from previous games or events, so they don't have the "muscle memory" to adjust quickly. Even something as simple as "stepping off the curb without breaking your ankle" requires the brain to remember how to hold the foot, how to shift weight, how to balance with the rest of the body. Without sleep, we're walking disaster areas.

Reaction times for motor skills increase. That means that for something like shifting lanes or avoiding a deer, your muscles aren't responding as quickly. You've lost the automatic memory, and that means you get into accidents.

Recalling things like dance routines also becomes harder. Without sleep, you lose your place, you can't match your moves to the rhythm, your motions get less fluid, and you become clumsier.

If you want your children to excel at dance, sports, art, or music, or even if you want them to become safe drivers, they need to sleep so that they have that "muscle memory" intact and somewhere they can use it.

Runaway Emotions

The toddler throws herself on the floor and starts sobbing over something small—a wrong shaped cracker, a broken banana, or a different cup than she was expecting. "Uh, oh," mom says, "looks like someone needs a nap!"

We all recognize how sleep affects emotions in small children. What we don't realize is that sleep loss affects adult emotional control too. People who aren't sleeping feel everything *more,* and they react more strongly to it, just like a toddler at naptime.

No Shades of Gray

A sleep-deprived person loses their ability to see normal events in a neutral light.

Think of all the little things that can go wrong on a quick trip to the store. The cart you choose may have a squeaky wheel. They may be out of the item you normally buy, so you have to buy a different one. There could be a line at the checkout because the person in front of you has to try multiple cards to find one that works. As you're returning to your car, someone might drive too fast through the parking lot—they might have hit you if you hadn't been paying attention!

As a well-rested person, you shrug these little things off. You get in the car, drive home, and the day goes on normally.

Without sleep, the brain latches on to the frustrations. Suddenly everything is proof that other people, or the universe itself, are out to get you. Everything is terrible. Everything is awful. You are sad or furious, just like that toddler.

Stuck on the Negative

Lack of sleep also causes excessive rumination, where you keep thinking about the bad things over and over. You can't just ignore the lady in line. Your brain gets stuck in a groove.

She's rude. She's inconsiderate. She's wasting your time. Your day was already terrible, and she's making it worse. Look at her; she doesn't even care. She enjoys holding up the line. She's a terrible person. She's ruining everything …

The more you ruminate, the angrier and angrier you get. This is a huge problem because sleep is also involved in impulse control.

Lashing Out

Toddlers are still learning emotional control. So whenever they have big feelings, they meltdown. As adults, we've learned to bite our tongue, take deep breaths, and count to ten, or wait and gripe later. Unfortunately, when we haven't slept, it's much harder to do these things.

Instead, we lash out. We might yell at the woman in line or be rude to the cashier. We might scream and pound on the hood of the car in the parking lot. Or we may take the bad mood home and yell at our families. Losing sleep doesn't just make us miserable. It makes everyone around us miserable, and it makes it harder for us to connect with them and for them to connect with us. It eats away at the relationships that make us who we are.

Putting it all together

So, what does it look like when you or someone you love is sleep-deprived over a long time, instead of just a single bad night? Your child or spouse might be crankier than they used to be. They're prickly and unable to let little things slide. They're alienating people and have more trouble at school or work.

Since everything is awful and they're stuck on negative thoughts and emotions, they may get more anxious or even depressed. They can't see good or neutral things anymore, so they have no hope. They've lost that fresh, happy, optimistic feeling that comes with a new day. If they can't get screened and treated, the mental health issues may begin to mask the underlying sleep issue so that it's harder to diagnose what's really wrong with them.

Complicated by Antidepressants

You'll notice that many of the effects of sleep loss on the brain look a lot like the symptoms of depression. Here's where things can get complicated. Many anti-depressants interfere with sleep, and especially the REM sleep we need to be socially aware, outgoing, and level-headed. If you put a patient with underlying sleep issues on an antidepressant, the drug may actually make their issues, and thus their depression, worse.

In fact, people whose depression is caused by sleep issues are often diagnosed with "treatment-resistant depression." Drugs and therapy don't work on them because the depression isn't caused by a brain chemical imbalance or a history of trauma. It's caused by not sleeping, and until you can get the sleep right, you can't fix the depression.

If you're newly presenting with depression, ask for bloodwork and a sleep study as part of the diagnostic process. Physical health has a huge impact on mental health, and sleep, especially, has huge effects that we often overlook.

Sleep Keeps You Sane

Doctors have known that there was a connection between mental illness and sleep loss for centuries, but they weren't sure which condition came first. Until the early twenty-first century, most psychologists believed that mental illness caused sleep loss—that not sleeping well was a symptom of the underlying illness.

In the last two decades, experiments have proven that, in many cases, the sleep deficit comes first. So, when you're sleeping poorly, due to breathing issues, restless legs, some other underlying issue, or even just because your schedule is a mess, you start having the emotional control issues that we just covered. As time goes on and you go longer and longer without sleep, those issues grow to the point where they can become a diagnosable mental illness.

For instance, in up to 20% of depression cases, OSA causes the depression. If you know someone with depression that doesn't respond to treatments, have them screened for OSA. Proper treatment that solves their underlying problem could turn their life around. Obstetricians now understand that sleep also plays a role in post-partum depression. The less sleep a new mother gets, the more likely she is to need depression medication. In teens, 69% of those who develop depression have sleep issues first. Bad sleep causes depression and may play a major role in the increase in depression in the US.

Sleep issues also play a role in bipolar disorder. A person whose illness is usually controlled well with medications can trigger a manic episode by skipping sleep. And sleep even affects less common disorders. In a British study of people with mental illness, CBT that improved sleep didn't just reduce anxiety and depression. It also improved symptoms like hallucinations and paranoia.

In identical twin studies, sleep quality affected whether a twin developed mental illness. Twins who slept well often remained mentally healthy, while their siblings who skipped out on sleep ended up needing treatment for mental illness. While not everyone has a genetic predisposition to mental illness, the evidence is clear: if you miss out on sleep or sleep poorly for a long time, it can take a serious toll on your mental health.

Social Skills Depend on Sleep

How are your social skills? Can you talk to the bank tellers or the cashier at the store? Or are you afraid to engage with strangers?

While some social preferences come from our personalities, a big chunk of our social skills come from sleep. When you deprive a person of good sleep over a long period of time, they lose their ability to navigate social interactions.

Your social skills depend on how much sleep you got the night before seeing people. People who don't get enough sleep report that they're very lonely. They feel anxious around other people, and in experiments, they are jumpier and afraid to let strangers near them. They avoid engaging with strangers, so they can't smile and chat with the stranger in line.

Sleep also predicts how other people respond to you. In experiments, the same person was rated "socially attractive" or "socially repulsive" depending on whether they'd had a good night's sleep before. When we're not sleeping well, something about our faces and our movements clues other people into it, and they avoid us. This can start a loneliness and anxiety feedback loop since other people's reactions reinforce your own sense that you are anxious and don't want to engage.

Finally, sleep impacts your ability to collaborate with other people at work and school. You feel less sociable, you have less emotional control, and you see neutral things as negative. You're no longer a good partner, and your career or school life suffers because your social skills suffer.

The good news is that even one night of good sleep can restore your social skills and change how other people see you. But if you or someone you love is feeling increasingly isolated and unable to reach out, poor sleep may be part of the problem.

Bad Habits Get Harder to Break

What are habits? They're chunks of actions that amount to one complex routine. For instance, someone who smokes doesn't just have a "smoking habit." Their habit includes going outside to a smoking area, opening the box, taking out a cigarette, lighting it, smoking it, putting it out in the ashtray, and going back inside. When you perform the first action in a habit, it's like you've gotten on a train, and you can't get off until it's reached the next station.

Forming new habits is hard because until you've completed a "chunk" many times, you have to think about each step and will yourself to complete it. Meanwhile, old habits are effortless. You go through the motions without even having to think.

When you get less sleep, it's harder to form new habits and harder to break old ones. Your emotional control is gone, so you can't force yourself through the steps in a new habit. Meanwhile, sleep loss dials up your reliance on existing habits, so your old habits become your default, and you just can't stop.

Without sleep, it's harder for addicts to give up drugs or alcohol. It's harder to start a new exercise program. It's harder to stop biting nails. The day happens on autopilot.

This is especially awful since the first-line advice for many people with sleep problems is "practice better sleep hygiene." This means creating new habits that support good sleep at the *very time* when your brain is least able to make new habits. So we tell you, "turn off the screens at 8:00 p.m.," but you're in the habit of playing mindless games or scrolling social media to wind down when you're tired. You literally don't have the brainpower to follow the advice you need to improve your sleep because you need sleep to follow the advice.

Looking for Food in All the Wrong Places

A sleepless brain doesn't just affect your mental state. Since the brain controls things like hormones, self-control, and movement, going without sleep also plays havoc with your body. For instance, getting less than seven to nine hours of good sleep at night will change how much you eat and which foods you crave.

Ellie was 58 years old when she switched to our practice. We immediately noticed the signs of jaw-clenching and tooth grinding. These can be symptoms of OSA and are also terrible for your teeth.

We fitted her with an appliance that both protected her teeth and repositioned her jaw to keep her airways clear. A year later, she'd lost 65 pounds. She had the energy to cook healthy, eat healthy, and exercise. She felt amazing, better than she had in at least twenty years.

So, she dragged her husband in to see us, against his will. He was sure he was fine and that she was exaggerating how bad his snoring was. We screened him, referred him for a sleep study, and, sure enough, he also had OSA.

He chose an oral appliance as well and also began to lose weight. Now, several years later, both are in excellent health. They have the energy to bike and swim and hike, and they can volunteer and be active in the community. It's incredible to see what a huge difference improving sleep has made in their lives.

When people sleep less than seven hours, their hormones that regulate hunger get out of sync. They consume more calories than they do when they're well-rested, even though they're tired and less active. The types of calories they consume also change. At a buffet, a well-rested person will eat a mix of fruit, veggies, protein, and maybe a few sweet or salty things, but not too many. A sleep-deprived person consumes many more calories, and the extra calories all come in the form of sweet and salty foods. So, without sleep, you eat more, and you eat a less balanced diet overall.

The situation gets even worse when someone is at home instead of at a buffet. Then, the craving for sugar, salt, and calories combines with mental and physical exhaustion. You crave unhealthy foods, and you gravitate to easy foods that don't take self-control or complex routines to prepare. Suddenly, cookies, chips, and ice cream seem like a fine dinner.

It only takes five days of reduced sleep for a person's new eating habits to result in weight gain. And, unless they fix the sleep issues, they don't have the mental resources to change habits, make healthier choices, and start exercising. Too little sleep quickly becomes too many calories and too much weight that won't come off no matter what you try.

How much money are you spending trying to lose weight when the key piece of the puzzle could be your sleep?

The Pain of Poor Sleep

Sleep also plays a big role in pain, how we feel it, and how we live with it. People with chronic pain often complain that pain keeps them from sleeping. They'll often sit up on the couch and zone out with the television because being in bed just hurts too much. They need a distraction from the pain so they can sleep.

However, less sleep actually makes the pain worse. Over time, getting too little sleep or bad sleep can cause chronic pain. Recent studies have confirmed that, while people who suffer from pain blame their poor sleep on the pain, the causality goes the other way. Bad sleep gives you chronic pain.

After just *one* night of reduced sleep, your brain changes how you experience pain. The areas for feeling pain become more active and more sensitive, so everything hurts more. The areas responsible for ignoring and soothing pain become less active, so you also can't ignore pain or recover as quickly. Without good sleep, life is painful.

Joint pain and headaches are especially common after a bad sleep. And when your joints hurt, it's harder to move. You just want to sit in a chair. Then, you're not tired the next night, and pretty soon, you're spiraling into chronic pain.

Sleep researchers do have good news, however. Healthy, high-quality sleep has a huge impact on pain. Matthew Walker, one of America's most influential sleep researchers, calls sleep "a natural analgesic." Good sleep can cure your pain.

A word of warning: Often, people in pain will resort to alcohol or sleep drugs to help them get to sleep despite the pain. However, since these chemicals interfere with the work of sleep, using them to blunt the pain at bedtime could set you up for even more pain the following day. If you have chronic pain, try to use natural ways of relaxing and soothing pain before bed so that you maximize your brain's pain-fighting potential.

Sick of Being Sleepless

The cascade of events that starts with a sleepless brain even affects your immune system. When you don't sleep, some parts of your immune system are suppressed, and some parts get cranked into high gear. For instance:

- **Tumor-killing cells are suppressed.** Normally, the immune system has cells whose job it is to find and kill tumor cells. These killer cells patrol the body, looking for the beginnings of tumors- cells with so many mutations that they lose their brakes and replicate over and over non-stop. If you don't sleep, you have fewer tumor-killers in the system, and so they're more likely to miss defective cells, and you're more likely to get cancer.

- **Viruses can flare-up.** Do you have cold sores? People with cold sores get flare-ups when they're not sleeping. So do people with a history of mononucleosis. The viruses that are normally kept in check by your immune system can start multiplying and cause a flare when poor sleep suppresses your immune system.

- **Vaccines are less effective**. Poor sleep affects your immune system's ability to recognize new diseases too. If you get vaccinated during a run of poor sleep, the vaccine can be up to 50% less effective. If you're not sleeping well, you're not as immune as you think you are.

- **You're more vulnerable to new infections, like colds, strep, and flu.** It's not just vaccines. A sleep-deprived immune system is more vulnerable to all sorts of diseases. Your mother probably told you that when you're "run down," you're more likely to get sick, and she was right. The longer you go without several nights of good sleep, the sicker you'll get.

- **You're more prone to autoimmune disorders.** Paradoxically, while your sleep-deprived immune system can't fight off outside invaders, it's more likely to increase inflammation and turn on your own body. Studies suggest that if someone is prone to autoimmune issues, a run of bad sleep can be the trigger that starts the disease process.

If you notice you're getting sick a lot more than you used to or having trouble kicking infections, bad sleep may be a part of the problem. It's worth getting screened to see if you can improve your immune system.

So many of us chug along on bad sleep. Our brains are struggling to function well, and we blame ourselves. We're spacey; we're lazy; we're weak; we're sickly. But, now that you've seen how a lack of good, restorative sleep injures the brain, you can see that, in many cases, it's not a moral problem; it's a medical problem. Fix the sleep, and you can fix many of the problems associated with poor sleep.

In the next two chapters, I'll share some profiles about what untreated sleep disorders like OSA or UARS look like in children and adults. If you see people you recognize in those stories, it's time to book a sleep screening with your dentist or physician.

The Take-Aways

- When you don't sleep, you lose the ability to learn and solve problems.
- Without sleep, you can't form new memories, so you lose chunks of your life.
- Skipping sleep makes it harder to complete multi-step tasks and leads to big, and sometimes dangerous, mistakes.
- You get clumsier as your motor memory gets impaired from lack of sleep. This can be a mild annoyance, resulting in stubbed toes around the house, or a major crisis if you're driving and get into a crash.
- Less sleep means less emotional control, a more negative outlook, and worse social skills.
- Bad habits are impossible to break without adequate sleep.
- Being sleepless changes your cravings and leads to unhealthy behaviors.

Try This

Track your sleep for two to three weeks while also keeping track of how many times you lose your temper each day. Do you see a connection?

Things to Think About

- Where do you feel fuzzy-headed or out of step in your life?
- What bad habits do you wish you could break?
- What new things do you wish you had the energy to learn?
- Are any of your kids having trouble with school or emotions?

6

When Your Child Isn't Sleeping: Profiles of Sleep Disordered Breathing (SDB) in Children and Teens

It can be hard to notice the signs of OSA in kids because every kid is so different. When you're used to a set of behaviors, you can just start thinking of them as your kid's personality. And since kids don't always react like adults to being very tired, it can be hard to pin down the problem. Also, many symptoms of OSA in children look like other conditions like learning disabilities or ADHD. And OSA can aggravate underlying issues, so you might blame behavior on the diagnosis, not the sleep breathing.

If you read one of these profiles and it sounds like your kid, or if bits and pieces of all of them sound like your kid, don't feel guilty. We all miss things. That's why we take our kids to see professionals! The important thing is that once you suspect your child has sleep breathing issues, you get them screened and get referrals to the appropriate specialists for diagnosis. You don't have to know everything. The important thing is that when you suspect something is wrong, you get help.

Emma the Lazybones

Everyone knew Emma was a lazy child. At home, on weekends, she'd flop on the couch, slack-jawed and open-mouthed as she played video games. If you turned off the screens, she whined. "I'm bored. There's nothing to do." Her parents would send her out to run and play with the neighborhood kids, but Emma would just sit on the front stoop, randomly doodling with sidewalk chalk and waiting to be allowed back inside.

On the soccer field, she got tired quickly. When everyone else ran, Emma stopped and walked, complaining all the way. She seemed to prefer being on the bench. When she got put in a game, she just stood there, barely paying attention to the game. She didn't even get excited when her team scored a goal. Emma was never excited about anything, and she was always bored.

At school, Emma spent a lot of time with her head on her desk. She didn't complete assignments or answer questions. The teachers had to drag her through everything. Emma was just lazy. She was even lazy about toileting, her mother confided. At eight years old, Emma still wet the bed almost every night. She had to wear pullups and couldn't go to slumber parties. It was like it was too much effort for her to wake up and walk to the bathroom in the middle of the night.

In many ways, Emma is a classic type of sleep-deprived child. Her parents and teachers are used to her behavior and assume she has control over it. But really, this child is just exhausted.

She's flopped on the couch or the front stoop because she literally doesn't have the energy to get up and do something else. She can drift in and out of sleep while playing her video games or watching TV, and she can't stay awake. This exhaustion shows up during school, outside in the yard, and during sports.

This is a child who is too tired to learn, play, or make friends. Every day she's too exhausted to function is a day full of missed opportunities. And because Emma is at an age where kids are supposed to be learning at a rapid rate, she's falling further and further behind.

The open-mouthed posture is because she hasn't developed good nasal breathing skills. This is often due to tongue-tie and high palate, untreated allergies, or chronic sinus infections. Mouth breathing irritates the throat, tonsils, and adenoids and can cause sleep-disordered breathing. Then, the SDB means that the child isn't getting good sleep, so the allergies and sinus infections are even worse. Parents and teachers often associate a slack-jawed posture with laziness or a lack of intelligence, but in reality, it is a huge red flag that a child isn't sleeping well.

Finally, the bed-wetting. Children have smaller bladders, and SDB causes microarousals. They wake up enough to catch their breath and feel the urge to urinate, but they're not all the way awake, so they don't wake up enough to get out of bed and use the restroom. Paradoxically, kids with a lot of microarousals LOOK like really deep sleepers. Nothing wakes these kids up. Having to use the bathroom, alarm clocks, smoke alarms. They can even vomit in their sleep and never seem to stir.

It's not because they're good sleepers. It's because they're terrible sleepers. Microarousals take their toll, they never really do the work of sleep, and so their bodies don't want to wake up because they've been almost waking up every few moments all night long.

SDB takes a horrible toll on these kids because they can't control their behavior. They don't know they're wetting the bed. They're genuinely exhausted and often in pain. Every day is a struggle, but often adults assume that it's a discipline issue, not a health issue. So you have kids internalizing the message that they're stupid, lazy, and babyish when, really, they're just not sleeping.

Emma, and kids like Emma, need help. With appropriate screening and exams by the relevant professionals, we can give these kids the energy they need to wake up, move, and learn.

Liam the Tornado

Liam never stopped moving. His parents were exhausted. His pre-school teachers were exhausted. The kid was just a constant whirlwind of flailing limbs and running mouth. When his parents took him to church, he'd flip and flop and kick and roll around the pew. His mother felt like she was fighting a battle the whole time.

On the playground, he was out of control. He'd run up to kids, poke them, and yell "TAG!" and then run off. If they didn't follow, he'd keep going back and poking and yelling until the other kids lashed out and hit him or ran crying to their mothers. And he didn't seem to improve with age.

He couldn't sit still to eat. He'd pick at his food, jump up, run around, grab a bite, wander off. "It's like he's still a toddler," his mom told his first-grade teacher. She had a lot of conversations with the teacher that year since Liam was a disaster in the classroom. He'd jump out of his seat, shout out comments, and act like a class clown. He was constantly picking fights with bigger boys and coming home bruised. His mouth ran constantly.

At home, he still moved a lot, and he was always bumping into things. Video games were the only thing that could get him to stay in one space for a bit. As bedtime approached, his mood would fall apart. He cried and shrieked every night, almost like a baby with colic. "It's like he's not even in his body," his mom complained. "His mind is just gone."

Liam even moved in his sleep. He still had night terrors at least two or three times a week, and he talked in his sleep so much that he couldn't share a room with his younger brother. He thrashed all night, too. In the morning, his mom would walk in to wake him and find him in a tangle of sweat-soaked sheets. But then he was up and running again. Maybe it was ADHD. He was in line for an evaluation, but there was a nine to twelve-month wait, and his parents were worried about how he was falling behind in school and couldn't make friends. Plus, they were exhausted and needed a break.

Believe it or not, Liam's symptoms scream sleep-disordered breathing just as much as Emma's do. Not all kids give in to the exhaustion and just fall asleep. Some kids try to fight the tired feeling, and the way they do it is by staying in a constant state of overstimulation.

For a kid like Liam, constant motion and talking is how he stays awake. If he lets his brain and body grow quiet, he might nod off, but he doesn't want to miss anything at home or school. So, instead, he becomes a tornado of activity, wearing out all the adults around him and irritating all the other kids.

Since sleep loss also affects his ability to control his emotions and read social cues, he can't make friends. He alienates other kids. He feels lonely and unconnected, so he goes after bigger kids like a little dog nipping at a big dog's heels. At some level, he knows it's not working, and he's not making friends, but he craves stimulation, and getting chased and hit by a bigger kid gives him a rush that keeps him going.

So, what are some clues that this sensory-seeking behavior is sleep-related rather than plain old ADHD or sensory issues? For one, the bedtime meltdowns. This is a really tired kid, but he's also fighting sleep. For some reason, he has negative associations with sleep, and that's common for kids with SDB. Their brain associates sleep with "almost suffocating over and over all night long," and so there's fear attached to sleeping.

Secondly, the night terrors. These can be linked to developmental or neurological issues, but they can also be caused by SDB, as the repeated drops in oxygen levels trigger panic attacks. The sleep talking and tossing and turning and sweating also point to some sort of sleep issue. This isn't normal sleep behavior.

Liam may have other issues affecting his behavior as well, but as part of the diagnostic process, his physician should rule out sleep issues. And, on a positive note, it is often possible to get a referral and get seen for suspected sleep issues very quickly. Getting any sleep issues diagnosed and treated now will also ensure he gets a more accurate diagnosis when he finally gets to see the developmental psychology team.

Celina the Anxious

Celina had always been a good student. She got A's effortlessly, and her teachers loved her. She wasn't a great athlete, but she tried hard. She got along with her classmates and teammates and always had nice words for everyone. Her only weird quirk was that she frequently complained of headaches first thing in the morning. Her mother assumed it was dehydration or just not being a morning person, and usually, by the time the school bus came, Celina was fine.

That all changed when Celina hit ninth grade. She was still doing fine in school, but her home life was terrible. She cried almost daily and would have screaming fits complaining that her work was too hard, she couldn't do it, it was wearing her out, and she didn't have time for anything but homework. She started to withdraw from her old friends. Her parents chalked it up to hormones and tried to weather the storm of Celina's big feelings. After all, school couldn't be that hard—Celina still had straight A's.

Things were even worse in tenth grade. Celina worried all the time, even though she still did well in her classes. Driver's ed was a disaster. She cried and panicked every time she got behind the wheel. "I can't do this," she explained over and over. "I never remember how. Practicing doesn't help. I can't do it." Celina's parents were worried. Could she have anxiety? They made an appointment to talk to their pediatrician.

At the doctor, Celina explained that she was just so tired and always in a fog. She kept up in all her classes, but it was really hard. Other kids didn't have this much trouble focusing, and by the end of the day, she was wrecked. And yes, she still had a headache every morning; she just figured no one cared.

Celina's parents were shocked when the doctor referred her to an ENT. They had literally never realized there could be something physically wrong with their child. She didn't act sick, after all, and her grades were fine.

Celina was an incredibly bright girl, so no one noticed her sleep problems for years. SDB may have been keeping her from reaching her potential, but since she was doing OK and a pretty undemanding kid, no one noticed. High school was the perfect storm, however. She still wasn't sleeping well, and the shift in teen circadian rhythms meant she had less opportunity to sleep. She had to master more material—school ramps up in difficulty as kids get older, and learning to drive is a whole new set of skills.

Celina knew she couldn't keep up. Lack of sleep was impacting her self-control, focus, and ability to learn. Her anxious meltdowns were a cry for help. She was anxious because she was struggling when no one else around her was.

By getting her sleep issues treated, Celina was able to start the day with a clear head for the first time in her life. Her parents were sad that they'd missed the symptoms for so long, but it's good that they got her help. Kids like Celina, whose sleep issues cause them to struggle in high school, often crash and burn once they hit college and work gets harder once again. The problem isn't a lack of intelligence or self-discipline. It's that they finally hit the point where their sleep-impaired brains can't keep up.

Always-Sick Henry

Henry looked like a sturdy child. He'd had a normal birth, seemed to be growing OK, and was generally pretty happy and sociable. The thing was, Henry was ALWAYS sick. If there was a flu going around, Henry got it. RSV? Expect a week of croup, even in elementary school? Strep? You betcha! He just seemed to have no immune system. Even mild colds that barely affected the rest of his siblings gave Henry a fever and a few days lying on the couch, feeling awful.

He'd been screened for asthma multiple times, but he didn't have it. He didn't seem to have any allergies. He snored, but everyone figured it was just because he was small and that he'd grow out of it. Henry did tend to mouth-breathe a lot because of the constant illness. Often his nose was just too stuffy to use.

As time went on, missing out on so many things was starting to have an impact on his life. He always had make-up work at school. He missed too many sports practices to play. His parents wouldn't let him go to birthday parties or playdates during flu and cold season because he just got sick too easily. One kid with a runny nose and Henry would be out of school for a week. His parents just couldn't risk another illness and more time out of work. Instead, they just waited, hoping he'd grow out of it. After all, no one had been able to find anything really wrong with their son. He was just sort of sickly.

When a child isn't getting good sleep, they tend to get sick more. And the mouth-breathing in response to illness can start a downward spiral. So, Henry gets yet another cold and spends the night alternating between snoring and mouth breathing.

The nose is essential to good breathing. It warms the air, humidifies it, and screens out particles that can damage your lungs. So, when Henry is mouth-breathing, he's sending cold, dry air full of irritants right down his windpipe and into his lungs.

What do you think happens next? The tonsils and adenoids get irritated and swell. His throat gets dry and scratchy too. His lungs get irritated. He can't breathe as well, so he doesn't sleep as well. That means his immune system takes a hit. He's more vulnerable to the next virus that comes around, and airways and lungs are irritated and more vulnerable to the next infection too.

This cycle repeats night after night. As soon as Henry's worn-down immune system clears one infection, he catches another. But no one can give him a good diagnosis because the underlying issue isn't asthma or allergies or anything. It's that he can't breathe at night, so he can't sleep.

For a kid like this, a consult with a pediatric ENT can be life-changing. Getting the right combination of interventions to get breathing right and support nasal breathing instead of mouth breathing means that the child finally gets a good night of sleep. And once the sleeping is better, the immune system gets better too. Kids like Henry deserve a shot at a normal life, and they miss out when we write them off as "just sickly."

Isaiah the Space Cadet

Isaiah was a nice kid, but he wasn't all there. In the morning, his mom had to walk him through every step of getting dressed. "Are you wearing pants? OK, go get your pants. Isaiah, where are your shoes?" He tried to comply, but the moment there was any distraction, it was like he was somewhere else.

At school, he'd forget to take his coat off. Or he'd forget that he was supposed to be working on math, and start doodling instead. He talked to his friends during lunch and forgot to eat. "You only have five minutes left, Isaiah," the aide would say, "and you haven't even touched your sandwich." Once, he was so distracted he forgot to come in from recess. When the class filed into their seats, the teacher noticed he was missing and had to go find him. He wasn't mischievous or defiant. He was just a space cadet.

Isaiah's mom met the bus every day. She had to, or he might forget to get off and ride clear to the county lot before anyone noticed. The other kids started making fun of him for how he could never focus. His mom and dad worried as they talked him through every step of every task. How would he ever survive adulthood? The child needed constant supervision to do something as simple as brushing his teeth or changing into pajamas.

He was otherwise smart and chatty. He remembered what he heard or read. He had lots of ideas about things, and he was pretty funny when he wanted to make a joke. But it was like his brain was completely unconnected from his body. Could he have ADHD or ASD?

Isaiah may have underlying issues, but can you spot the big red flag here? Remember how we talked about how sleep loss makes people forget where they are in complex tasks? For a child, things like getting dressed, unpacking and eating lunch, or brushing teeth *are* complex tasks. They haven't done them enough to be able to do them on autopilot. That means that if a child's working memory is impaired, they'll often appear to be unfocused, spacey, and unable to complete "simple" tasks (that aren't actually that simple).

The pediatrician should complete a sleep screening and rule out sleep difficulties as part of Isaiah's diagnostic process. However, many practices still fail to screen all of their patients, even though the American Academy of Pediatrics has recommended routine screening at checkups for nearly two decades.

One reason that this screening is so important is that underlying learning, developmental, and behavioral disabilities can be made more severe by lack of sleep. When we get the sleep issues corrected, kids are more able to respond to interventions like occupational therapy. OT is hard work, so the brain needs sleep to give a child the full benefits.

No Shame in Asking for Help

Do you recognize your children, or children you know, in these examples? Because sleep breathing affects every system of the body, kids can react to SDB in many different ways. But the key thing to keep in mind is that these kids are not OK. They're not able to reach their potential. They're not healthy, and they're being set up for more serious health problems down the road if their sleep issues go untreated.

If you have a child who resembles the kids in this chapter, please, get them screened for sleep issues. The right interventions can help them in school, with their peers, and with their overall mood and health. If you don't address the underlying sleep issues, you'll end up with a long list of interventions that you tried and that didn't work very well or completely failed. Sleep is the foundation of everything else our kids do in a day.

The Take-Aways

- Many "bad kid" behaviors are actually "unwell kid" behaviors, and a lack of sleep can make a kid unwell.

- Kids have very little control over their schedules, so a kid who has sleep issues AND is a night owl is in especially bad shape.

- Symptoms of sleep disturbance in kids can look a lot like ADHD, anxiety, or learning disabilities. And when a kid with one of these conditions also has a sleep issue, it exacerbates their condition.

Try This

Keep a journal of your child's sleep and behavior. Track symptoms like snoring, waking, bedwetting, morning headache, coughing, and dark circles under their eyes. Then write down any behavior or learning issues. Is there a connection between the severity of their sleep symptoms on a given night and their school issues the next day?

Things to Think About

- Which of your child's problematic behaviors may be sleep-related?
- How is their behavior over school breaks, when they can get more sleep?
- Has your child been evaluated for sleep issues yet? How soon can you set up an evaluation?

Adults Need Sleep Too —What it Looks Like When They Aren't Getting It

Kids are lucky. They have parents and teachers watching them, worrying about them, and looking out for them. So even though it might take a while for someone to pinpoint what's wrong, when kids are having problems, they have many people to advocate for them.

But what about adults? If you snore, does anyone notice? Maybe you live alone, or maybe your spouse goes to bed first and is a heavy sleeper. If you're having health issues, is there someone in your life to tell you to get checked out, or do you just chalk everything up to age and stress?

The following profiles show the lives of typical adults with undiagnosed sleep breathing problems like OSA or UARS. Do you see yourself in them? Do you find yourself saying, "Well, sure, but doesn't everyone do that?" If you do, check in with your dentist or physician and ask for a sleep breathing screening. It's not just your children who deserve attention and care. You deserve to have your sleep problems diagnosed and treated too.

Allen's Story

Really, it was the commute that was killing him, thought Allen. Lately, he just couldn't stay awake on the road. It was an hour to work, and an hour home, and he found himself drifting off between towns and drifting across the lanes of traffic.

Luckily, he'd recently started craving sugar. He hadn't been a soda person before, but now a huge gas station cup of Mountain Dew hit the spot. The sugar tasted great these days, and between that and the caffeine, he was sort of doing OK.

When he got home at night, he'd go straight to his chair and nod off before dinner. His wife kept complaining that he was gaining weight and snoring, but what did she expect? He was in his fifties now; it was all downhill from here. He should replace his morning Mountain Dew with an unsweet iced tea, he guessed. But somehow, when he was standing there, he always picked the pop. It called to him, and he could always start being healthier tomorrow.

His phone beeped. His doctor had texted him something about wanting him to come in and discuss bloodwork. Good grief. Why was his body falling apart so quickly? At this rate, how much longer would he be able to keep working?

Allen has a lot of risk factors for OSA here. Most importantly, he has excessive daytime sleepiness. Falling asleep while you're driving is a huge red flag that you're not getting enough high-quality sleep. A healthy adult should be able to tolerate an hour-long drive without excessive drowsiness. And Allen is falling asleep for long enough to drift across lanes. Again, this is not OK. His sleep issues are putting his life, and the lives of other drivers, in immediate danger. This symptom alone is enough reason to get checked out.

But Allen also has other symptoms that point to OSA. His cravings have changed recently, and he's suddenly got a sweet tooth where he didn't have one before. Lack of sleep could be causing him to crave high-sugar, high-salt foods, and beverages. His self-control has also taken a hit. He can't bring himself to make a healthier choice.

Finally, we have the physical symptoms. He's snoring, he has weight gain, and he is starting to have problems with his bloodwork. This is a man who needs a sleep screening and, most likely, a sleep study. The hard part is convincing people like this that their problem is not simply "getting old or not trying hard enough" and that they are worth the time and trouble of a sleep study.

Theresa's Story

Theresa was just draggy and achy all the time. She chalked it up to being the single mother of a very active eight-year-old girl. Charlee was active, sassy, and went full tilt from dawn to dusk, so anyone would be tired. Still, Theresa tried hard to live a healthy life. She didn't buy treats—she knew that she'd binge if there were cookies or ice cream in the house, and the easiest time to say "no" was on the grocery order. She and some of the girls from work took a 2-mile walk every day at lunch, so she stayed trim and in good shape.

She was just so, so sleepy. It made her cranky at bedtime with her daughter because she had trouble making it through the routine when she was so tired herself. Then she'd wake up multiple times a night, feeling like she was choking. Her sinuses always felt like they were on fire too, and in the morning, her mouth was so dry.

Theresa never considered that there might be something wrong until her family practice doctor wanted to do a sleep screen on Charlee. Theresa realized that she had many of the same symptoms. But how could she have a sleep disorder? She was careful about her health, and she wasn't overweight at all!

Theresa has a common misconception about sleep-disordered breathing—that it only affects the overweight. But while excess weight can cause OSA, untreated SDB can also eventually lead to weight gain. In Theresa's case, there's a good chance she has UARS—which is common in people who are at a healthy weight, but it can cause weight gain and progress to OSA if left untreated. Her constant exhaustion and achiness are big red flags here, as is her irritability. Something is interfering with her ability to be a great mom to her daughter, and that something is most likely poor sleep.

Many symptoms of UARS show up during a dental exam, for instance, a high palate or a pronounced overbite. Theresa may not be experiencing full apneas, where her breathing is completely blocked. However, if her airway is narrowed, she may still be struggling to breathe, waking up constantly, and missing out on the work of sleep. If she gets treated now, she might be able to avoid the progression that includes weight gain, health issues, and full-blown OSA.

Mark's Story

He couldn't remember when the downward spiral started. He'd been depressed and socially anxious, and he discovered that drinking made it possible to deal with people. He'd always had trouble sleeping, and the alcohol helped with that too. His job was incredibly irritating and demeaning. His knees started to go. He was gaining weight, and his blood pressure was sky high even though he didn't think he was drinking that much. Then, the infections started. "The Valley Crud," he called it. One sinus infection after another. Sore throat after soar throat. It got even harder to sleep, and so he drank more, hoping for at least a little bit of oblivion every night.

His sister finally convinced him to check into rehab. She'd come down for a visit and had been worried by how haggard he looked. The medical detox was hard, but not as hard as he'd expected, given the severity of his symptoms. A few weeks into the program, one night-clerk stopped him on his way to his room. "Your snoring is pretty terrible. Have you ever had a sleep test?"

The doctor declared that his OSA was off-the-charts bad. Listening to his medical history, the doctor was optimistic. "If you use the CPAP regularly, I think you'll find that many of the other problems take care of themselves." Mark couldn't believe it. How could something so simple have such a big effect on every part of his life?

Mark's alcohol issues can be very common in people with OSA. Often, repeated stop breathing experiences trigger insomnia because the brain no longer associates sleep with rest. People are depressed and anxious from the lack of sleep and become socially withdrawn.

As time goes on, an insomniac with OSA becomes more and more desperate for any downtime at all, even if it's not real sleep. So they turn to artificial sleep, in the form of sleep aids or alcohol. Their bodies fall apart, both from the drugs but also from lack of sleep. They're more irritable; they're sicker, everything always hurts.

Even worse, alcohol can make OSA worse. So the patient gets into a feedback loop. They can't sleep well, so they drink. They drink, so they can't sleep well. There's a cascade of bad effects that injures their mind and their body.

If they treat the addiction without spotting the underlying sleep problem, their chances of success aren't great. The same issues that drove them to drinking or drugs before are still there, and eventually, they'll give in to temptation because not sleeping takes a horrible toll on the mind, the body, and the will.

If you or a loved one struggles with alcohol, please get a sleep screening as part of your recovery processes. Improving your sleep increase your odds of success in recovery and change your life—and the lives of your friends and family.

Moira's Story

After baby number four, Moira couldn't lose the baby weight. She was tired all the time too, but most health care providers didn't take her seriously. "Of course, you're a bit tired! You have four kids!" "Have you tried losing weight? Exercise more and eat healthier, and you'll have more energy."

Moira gave up. This was her new, middle-aged, dumpy mom normal, she guessed. She kept trying to exercise and eat well, but the weight never came off. It was like her body had just forgotten how to lose weight. She was achy a lot of the time, and she was developing mild anxiety, but she kept pushing herself. But still, everyone felt the need to tell her to exercise and eat more vegetables. She was eating ten servings of fruits and veggies a day and only drank water and green tea! Moira began to withdraw and spend less time with other women. She felt like her weight made her a freak.

Her blood pressure kept rising, and her diastolic numbers were especially high. They seemed resistant to diet, exercise, or medication. Even worse, her most recent blood tests suggested that she might be prediabetic. Her thyroid and other biomarkers were fine, however. Friends suggested it might just be the stress of young children. Also, had she tried dieting and exercising to lose some weight?

When her youngest child entered kindergarten, Moira decided to make a big change in her life. She'd always been a great student, but she'd put her career and advanced education on hold so that she could raise the kids. Now she was going to go back, get her Master's, and reenter the workforce.

The problem was the brain fog. She couldn't learn anymore. Things no longer stuck in her head; she read more slowly, she looked at math from fifteen years before, and it no longer made sense. Plus, she kept nodding off during lectures. Was this early menopause? Was she out of practice? Had the children destroyed her brain? It was the school issues that caused Moira to talk to a new doctor, a woman around her age who also had several kids. And this was the first time in her life that Moira heard the words "obstructive sleep apnea."

Moira's story is a common one. When a middle-aged mom can't lose weight, a lot of her peers, and her physicians, tend to treat it as a moral issue. "Exercise more! Try harder! Eat better!" What they don't understand is that these women are already doing those things and not losing weight. The "calories in, calories out, have more self-control" method is failing them. Then, all their subsequent health problems get blamed on the extra pounds. But often, all of these issues are actually symptoms of a larger, underlying health problem, like a sleep issue.

For many mothers, it's difficult to get the symptoms of OSA taken seriously until you have an objective measure like grades or falling asleep at the wheel. And even then, physicians often write it off as "of course you're tired." Moira's case was helped because she could give a concrete example. "I fall asleep in lectures."

For you, it might be "I need a nap even if I sleep through the night," or "I can't unload the dishwasher without stopping to gather my strength," or "I don't have enough energy to take a short walk with my family, and I used to be able to hike for hours." If you're not sure if your sleepiness is excessive, consider using a screening tool like the Epworth Sleepiness Scale before you talk to your doctor, so you can give a clearer picture of how sleepy you are and how your exhaustion is affecting your daily life.

If Moira goes through the process to get diagnosed and treated for OSA, she can expect to see big changes in her life. First, her Master's work will get easier since her brain will be ready and able to learn again. Her hormone profile will change. She'll have less stress and anxiety. The steps that she's been taking to try to improve her health will finally have a chance to work because she'll have dealt with the underlying problem that's causing all of her body's systems to break down. Sleep is the key to a healthy, active middle age.

Getting Help

Again, if you recognize yourself in these stories, talk to someone who can help. Dentists and physicians can conduct sleep screenings, refer you to the necessary specialists, and help you start getting the sleep you need. The sooner you deal with your issues, the better. In the next chapter, we'll go into some of the long-term, often irreversible damage that comes from years or decades without enough high-quality sleep. So much of America's chronic illness can be traced back to poor sleep. And so many lives could be improved if we could get every single person screened on an annual basis.

The Take-Aways

- Falling asleep at the wheel is very dangerous. Treat it like a medical emergency.
- Untreated SDB can lead to big health issues down the road.
- Treat SDB early to prevent weight gain.
- Poor emotional control from bad sleep can start a cycle that leads to addiction.
- Brain fog is a sign that something is wrong.

Try This

Make a list of health problems that have gotten worse for you over the last decade. Could sleep be a culprit?

Things to Think About

- What are your most pressing health concerns?
- How many medications are you on? What are their side effects?
- Are you willing to see if improving sleep can improve your health markers?

Short on Sleep, Long on Problems— The Long-Term Consequences of Sleep Disordered Breathing

Up till now, we've talked about many of the immediate consequences of low-quality, interrupted sleep. Since microarousals keep your body from doing the work of sleep, after even one bad night, you feel mentally slow, emotionally raw, and physically ill. But, of course, no one goes to their physician about sleep difficulties after one bad night, or even after a few weeks of bad nights. For most people who suffer from SDB, years go by before they finally get the help they need.

In this chapter, I'll explain, in-depth, some of the long-term consequences of untreated SDB for adults and children. I hope that you'll realize that the longer you let SDB go without treatment, the worse the outcomes. You and your loved ones deserve prompt screening, diagnosis, and treatment for your sleep breathing issues. Putting off care can have disastrous consequences.

SDB and Alzheimer's Disease

Few diseases of aging are scarier than Alzheimer's Disease. If you've lost someone to it, you remember the pain of watching them lose chunks of themselves, lose the memories of their closest family, and become increasingly scared, angry, and confused. There are so many interventions that claim to reduce the risk of Alzheimer's or other forms of dementia—remember the Sudoku fad? But somehow, the link between SDB and Alzheimer's isn't as familiar as the advice like, "Drink fermented beverages!"

Research keeps finding new connections between SDB and Alzheimer's, and scientists have even found a plausible way in which untreated SDB could lead to Alzheimer's Disease as someone ages. Remember how, during the work of sleep, your body heals and grows? One function of sleep is to remove amyloid plaques from the brain. These are the same plaques that we find in the brains of people with Alzheimer's. OSA prevents the unbroken sleep you need to remove these plaques. In fact, the process of amyloid plaque build-up due to OSA follows the same pattern as plaque buildup due to Alzheimer's.

There seems to be a bidirectional relationship between sleep-disordered breathing and Alzheimer's. SDB can kickstart the Alzheimer's disease process, and then as the disease progresses, the Alzheimers increases the severity of the SDB, which then speeds the progression of Alzheimer's. More severe OSA, for instance, leads both to an earlier age of onset and a swifter progression of the disease.

There is some good news about SDB and Alzheimer's. Treatment can delay the onset of the disease and reverse some of the existing cognitive declines in patients with Alzheimer's. In a sleep lab, technicians can measure the number of times that a person's airway partially collapses (a hypopnea) or totally collapse (an apnea) during sleep. The number of full and partial collapses per hour is the Apnea-Hypopnea Index or the AHI for short. A person's AHI influences the age of onset and severity of cognitive impairment in Alzheimer's, with a higher AHI predicting earlier onset and faster progression of the disease. Treatments that reduce the AHI can give people more time before cognitive decline sets in, which translates to more years of health and more years out in the community, living an active life with friends and family.

If you're serious about preventing Alzheimer's for yourself or your family, set down the Sudoku for a moment, and make an appointment for a sleep screening. Treating SDB now can prevent irreversible damage down the road.

Type 2 Diabetes

According to the CDC, 10-20% of US adults will develop Type II Diabetes during their lives. In T2D, the cells of the body develop insulin resistance—it takes more and more insulin to "unlock" the cells so that they can take sugar out of the blood. Your cells need sugar for respiration and to repair themselves, so while your blood sugar goes up, your cells also die. Your body goes haywire because your blood sugar is sky-high, but your cells are starving. Eventually, your pancreas can't handle the load anymore, and you become insulin-dependent as well.

Because T2D can lead to so many health complications, it's important to avoid it. A healthy diet and exercise can prevent or reverse insulin resistance. But if you have SDB, these interventions won't be enough. That's because the trauma that your body is undergoing every night during sleep is creating the insulin resistance. Untreated SDB can lead to T2D and all the complications that go with it.

Not only does SDB lead to insulin resistance, but the severity of your issues can determine your risk for developing diabetes in the next five years. The lower your oxygen level during sleep, and the more apneas you have, the worse your blood sugar control and the more quickly you develop insulin resistance. Even if your treatment plan doesn't eliminate apneas and hypoxias, by improving your numbers, you improve your outcomes.

Without treatment, the combination of SDB and T2D can become deadly. The two conditions have a bidirectional relationship. That means that SDB makes T2D more severe, but one of the effects of T2D is increasing the severity of your SDB. You get in a feedback loop, spiraling out of control and adding complication upon complication.

The good news is that there is help. Patients with SDB and T2D who get treated for their sleep breathing issues see their blood sugar get easier to control. And with more sleep, it becomes easier to see results from eating healthy and losing weight. In fact, getting treatment for SDB can reverse your insulin resistance and prevent T2D or even send the disease into remission!

It's also important to recognize that this is not just an adult problem. Children with OSA can also develop insulin resistance, pre-diabetes, and T2D. We're seeing more and more children and teens coming in with what we used to consider a "disease of aging," and bad sleep is partly to blame. If these kids don't get treated, they can have a lifetime of blood sugar issues and damage to all the systems of their bodies because of the bad sleep they got when they were small.

While the number of studies showing these links keeps growing, many practices do not automatically screen pre-diabetic or diabetic patients for sleep breathing issues. So, if you haven't been screened in the last year, ask about sleep breathing. Don't stay silent or worry about bothering your care team. Your health is too important for that!

Janet, age 42, came into my office for a hygiene appointment and was updating her health history. In the last year, she'd gone from healthy to a whole mess of health issues. She was chalking the new cholesterol, blood sugar, and blood diagnoses up to "everything goes downhill after 40." But it wasn't a magic consequence of a few birthdays. Sleep apnea was driving that decline. When we got her diagnosed and treated, all of those worrying numbers reversed themselves. She was healthy again, without the need for medication or any intervention other than an oral appliance.

Heart Arrhythmias

Most of the time, we don't notice our hearts. They beat along regularly through the day, and we don't feel them or think about them. Have you ever had palpitations or arrhythmia? Have you felt like your heart skipped a beat? It's a terrifying feeling, isn't it? Suddenly you can't trust that your heart will keep going. You could drop dead at any moment. Your life is fragile, and your heart has just reminded you of that fact.

SDB has been linked to cardiac arrhythmias. People who have sleep breathing issues are two to four times more likely than their agemates to have issues with their heart rhythm, and the worse their breathing, the greater their risk of heart rhythm problems. Somewhere between 30 and 50% of people diagnosed with OSA also have arrhythmias.

Outcomes are even worse for people whose SDB occurs mostly during REM sleep instead of during NREM sleep. Cardioversion, shocking the heart back into the right rhythm, is often the first-line treatment for these patients. However, if their SDB remains untreated, cardioversion is more likely to fail. These are the patients who end up on a pacemaker for the rest of their lives.

The good news is that some of these rhythm issues can be reversed if the sleep breathing issues are caught early enough. The link between heart arrhythmia and OSA is strong enough that if you've been diagnosed with a heart arrhythmia, you should talk to your care team about possible sleep issues.

Obesity

Obesity can cause sleep apnea. But did you know that SDB can cause obesity? Many thinner adults don't have full-blown OSA, but they have UARS. This means that their airflow is restricted, their O2 sats drop during sleep, and they have microarousals, just like you see with sleep apnea. This affects their blood sugar levels and their hormones.

Because of SDB, these patients feel tired and draggy all day. They don't have the energy to exercise. They have to conserve their strength for things like work or childcare. They also have the cravings that go with skipped sleep. They eat more calories, and they eat more carbs and sugars. And their bodies are under stress from poor sleep, so they also gain weight from that. Eventually, the weight gain tips them into being overweight or obese, they accumulate fatty deposits on their tongue or fat in their necks, and the SDB advances to become OSA, which in turn contributes to further weight gain.

This same trend also occurs in kids. Untreated SDB at age five is correlated with obesity at age fifteen. It's socially, emotionally, and physically painful for a teen to be obese. It is very important to catch these kids early so that they can stay healthy throughout their childhood.

The best way to lose weight is not to gain it in the first place. Treating SDB early can prevent weight gain by helping your energy levels, will power, and cravings. "It's not that bad; I can live with it," really means "It's not that bad *yet*, I can live with it *right now*." But you have a long life ahead of you, and getting treated maximizes your chances for a healthy, active life.

Cancer

Cancer is another fear that haunts us all. Who hasn't watched a loved one suffer through diagnosis, radiation, and chemo? Who hasn't lost someone to this terrible disease? Our country spends so much time and effort on cancer prevention, yet it still takes a horrible toll. Could sleep-disordered breathing be an overlooked risk factor?

Recent research says yes. Studies around the world have turned up links between SDB and cancer. Early studies in mice seemed to show that OSA leads to more tumors, faster tumor growth, and more metastasis.

In humans, the link also seems clear. A recent study in Ontario looked at 30,000 patients and found that the more times a person stopped breathing in an hour, the higher their risk of developing cancer. There was a 15% increase for people who stopped breathing thirty times an hour. And the lowest blood oxygen levels, even without apneas, correlated with a 30% increase in cancer risk. Another recent study found that for women under sixty-five, OSA results in two to three times the cancer risk of women without sleep breathing issues.

SDB has been shown to increase the risk of colorectal cancer, lung cancer, kidney cancer, and melanoma (skin cancer). But, once again, treatment helps. Adhering to treatment plans dropped SDB patients' cancer risk compared to patients who didn't treat their sleep breathing issues. Treating sleep apnea doesn't just mean feeling better right now. It also means saving lives down the road.

Hypertension and SDB

According to the CDC, 45% of American adults have hypertension. The risk of developing high blood pressure goes up with age. Over time, uncontrolled hypertension can lead to heart failure, heart attacks, and strokes. High blood pressure is often referred to as a silent killer because it can damage hearts and blood vessels for years before someone's symptoms are bad enough to go to the doctor.

SDB plays a major role in your risk of developing hypertension. When the body can't do the work of sleep, damage to the heart and blood vessels doesn't get repaired. Over time, this begins to affect your blood pressure.

Poor breathing and microarousals also put extra stress on your cardiovascular system. In a healthy sleeper, blood pressure dips overnight. Your heart and blood vessels get a much-needed break. With SDB, the stress is constant. You're always "on." There's extra inflammation in your heart and blood vessels, too. This causes elevated blood pressure at night, and those highs carry over into the day.

In studies of adults with hypertension, 20 to 40% of them also had untreated OSA. When researchers looked at adults whose high blood pressure did not respond to medication, 70% of them had OSA. OSA can be a major factor in HBP, and without treating the underlying issue, it can be difficult to treat the blood pressure issues.

In the earlier stages of SDB in children and young adults, only the diastolic (bottom) blood pressure is elevated during the day. Over time, the systolic blood pressure rises as well. If you have diastolic blood pressure issues, and especially a high diastolic blood pressure that doesn't respond to medication, you should ask your medical team about a sleep screening.

Treatment for OSA can restore the nighttime dip in blood pressure. It can also lower daytime blood pressure. In kids, the drop is significant, and treatment can eliminate hypertension. In an adult, the results aren't as great. If you catch SDB before you develop hypertension, you can prevent it. But once the damage is done to your heart and blood vessels, it's not easily reversible.

Once high blood pressure develops, SDB treatments produce a very small drop in blood pressure, and sometimes these benefits can take up to a year of treatment before they show up. Early screening for and treatment of SDB is essential for preventing hypertension and its complications.

Autoimmune Disorders

Autoimmune disorders are something of a mystery. Often, they seem to come out of nowhere, triggered by an infection, stress, or some other event. Suddenly, your body is attacking itself, and most of your medication options have some pretty scary side effects. People have a genetic predisposition to them, but the onset seems to be a combination of genes and bad luck.

Sleep scientists have discovered that SDB can be a trigger for the onset of autoimmune disorders, perhaps because of the way it can trigger excessive inflammation. A University of Georgia team recently found that people with untreated SDB have unusual levels of cytokines compared to people without SDB and people with treated SDB.

Cytokines are part of the body's immune system. They cause inflammation, and they alert the body to the existence of invaders. If cytokines are released when there's not an infection, the immune system may attack healthy cells in the body instead. That can cause an autoimmune disorder, where the immune system attacks the body and causes damage.

The new findings explain something that Taiwanese scientists discovered in 2012: people with OSA are almost twice as likely to develop an autoimmune disorder than people without OSA. Diseases like rheumatoid arthritis and psoriasis are especially common in people who have a history of SDB and, especially, OSA.

Again, there is good news. In the most recent study, people who were treated for OSA have normal cytokine levels. If autoimmune disorders run in your family, it's especially important to get screened for issues with your sleep breathing. By correcting sleep breathing issues, you may be able to protect your health and avoid autoimmune disorders.

Atherosclerosis

Atherosclerosis, or hardening of the arteries, is a disease process that's part of heart disease. Over time your blood vessels become inflamed, swollen, and less flexible. They start to form plaques and narrow even further. Eventually, blood has trouble moving through them. They can become blocked or rupture, leading to a heart attack, stroke, or aneurysms.

Obstructive sleep apnea is associated with atherosclerosis, especially in the carotid arteries (some doctors call these the "widowmaker" arteries because blockage here often leads to sudden death from cardiac events). The interrupted sleep and oxygen loss of OSA kicks off an inflammation process. In some studies, as little as two weeks of intermittent low oxygen can start the attack on the walls of your blood vessels. Plaque formation is also worse with OSA because, without uninterrupted sleep, your body can't heal and clear out the plaques before they become a problem.

Scientists have also found that untreated OSA and high blood pressure together do twice as much damage as either one does on its own. The severity of the damage and the speed at which atherosclerosis progresses is related to the severity of OSA, and untreated OSA means that you're much more likely to die from a cardiac event.

Again, there is hope. Treatment for SDB can reverse some of the damage to your arteries, especially if you get treatment early in the disease progression. Again, so many of these "diseases of aging" are also "diseases of sleep breathing." Taking care of your airway issues can give you a healthier old age.

Heart Failure

Heart failure is another cardiac condition that seems to be directly related to sleep-disordered breathing. Some studies have found that between 47 and 81% of heart failure patients have sleep-disordered breathing. Once again, the relationship is bidirectional. SDB can cause heart failure, but the fluid retention common in heart failure can also increase the severity of sleep-disordered breathing.

In many studies, SDB can lead to heart failure even in patients who aren't overweight or obese. Patients with the "excessive sleepiness" subtype of SDB seem the most likely to develop heart failure, regardless of the number of apneas or hypoxias they have an hour.

OSA, in particular, predicts how likely someone is to die from heart failure. The more severe the OSA, the earlier the disease develops and the faster it progresses. Patients with OSA and HF together are more likely to die after a hospitalization.

Treatment for SDB can improve heart function and reduce the risk of death. Also, SDB treatment can improve energy levels and let patients exercise. This improves their quality of life and reduces their chances of death.

Stroke

Sleep-disordered breathing is a major risk factor for both TIAs and stroke. In fact, there's a growing consensus that anyone who suffers from a TIA should undergo a full OSA screening. In studies, 62% of TIA patients also have OSA. That's because TIAs are a warning that a major stroke is in your future. Twenty-five percent of people with

TIA have a second, major event soon after. And OSA is one thing that increases the odds of a poor outcome after a TIA.

Many TIA patients with OSA don't match the stereotypical OSA or stroke profile. They're younger than your typical stroke patient. They're not necessarily overweight. Many are careful about their diet, and they exercise frequently. If you know a fairly young, health-conscious person who seems to have had a TIA out of the blue, OSA may be a factor.

People with untreated SDB are twice as likely to have a stroke as people who have healthy sleep breathing. And if you stop breathing or have low oxygen more than thirty-six times an hour, you're three times as likely to have a stroke as someone without SDB. Snoring also seems to be related to stroke risk, independent of oxygen levels, and stop breathing incidents. One study found that the frequency, loudness, and pattern of snoring could accurately predict someone's stroke risk.

Patients who get diagnosed with SDB and comply with their treatment plan heal more quickly from the first event and prevent future strokes. In 2019, stroke was the fifth most common cause of death in the US. Treating SDB prevents strokes and saves lives.

Early Death

The physical problems caused by years of sleep-disordered breathing lead to an early death. The longer you live with untreated SDB, the sicker you'll be and the sooner you'll die. In large studies, severe OSA can lead to three to four times the death risk from all causes. It's not just heart issues or strokes. Untreated SDB means you're at greater risk for accidents at work and on the road. You're more likely to die in your sleep.

You're even more likely to die after surgery. Undiagnosed and untreated SDB leads to sudden, unexpected death after surgeries, often when a patient is on a regular care floor. This is because anesthesia and painkillers can affect muscle control and breathing. If you already had issues with sleep breathing, recovery from surgery could make you worse.

Many sedation medicines, like drugs in the benzodiazepine family, are contraindicated for OSA. Even very small doses of opioids can kill someone with untreated SDB, and the first twenty-four hours after surgery are the most dangerous for patients.

Surgeons are beginning to recognize the connection between sudden death and SDB, and many are starting to screen patients before surgery. However, thin patients or patients who don't experience daytime sleepiness often get missed. Untreated SDB kills.

It's not just physical problems

It's not just physical problems. Long-term SDB also has consequences for mental, social, and emotional health:

Educational Outcomes

Children with SDB miss out on learning, get worse grades, and score lower on cognitive assessments. Because education builds on what went before, over time, they fall further and further behind. They may miss out on educational opportunities or never reach their full potential because of their disease.

Children who have untreated SDB before the age of five are more likely to need special education services at age eight.

Career Problems

Untreated SDB affects careers. People with untreated OSA are more likely to be unemployed and to be fired or laid off multiple times over the course of their lives. They're more likely to be in low-wage, hourly jobs instead of in salaried jobs with benefits. They are more likely to end up on disability.

Untreated OSA leads to more workplace accidents, so people with it may gravitate to safer, less fulfilling, and lower-paying careers. It leads to "presenteeism," where people show up to work but are unable to complete tasks due to illness.

Financial Problems

The education and career problems that come with SDB lead to life-long financial problems. People with SDB are less likely to have jobs that provide good insurance, but they also use more medical care and have higher health costs. This makes it harder to save money. Because they are more accident-prone, they're likely to have higher car insurance rates and can't keep cars for as long. Throughout a lifetime, all the little costs of untreated SDB add up. SDB can make people poor.

Mental Health Issues

Remember how a single night without sleep can make you anxious, depressed, and socially withdrawn? Now take that one bad night and multiply it over weeks, or years, or decades. What do you think happens next?

Untreated SDB can lead to anxiety and depression, and the mental illnesses it causes are resistant to treatment. Over time, it can even lead to suicide attempts. Depression takes a toll on family and relationships too. SDB can isolate people and leave them without the supports they need to navigate life with a chronic illness.

The good news is that when depression and anxiety are caused by SDB, they can be cured very quickly by treatments that target SDB. Life isn't always going to be terrible. You're very tired, but there is help, and it's a pretty simple fix. SDB treatment can turn lives around because an open airway changes lives.

Now what?

I hope this section of the book has convinced you that SDB is a public health crisis and that it's a *treatable and preventable* crisis. Most people reading these pages will recognize themselves or someone they love because undiagnosed SDB is also very common. In the next section, I'll show you what steps you need to take to get screened, diagnosed, and treated for SDB. I'll also show you some of your treatment options. Not everything works for everyone, and you must find a treatment plan you can comply with. For now, I want you to remember: the long-term outlook for someone with untreated SDB is poor, but now that you know, you can get help, halt or reverse disease processes, and look forward to a longer, healthier life!

The Take-Aways

- SDB plays a role in many diseases of aging, including type II diabetes, Alzheimer's, and cardiovascular disease.
- Poor sleeping can shorten your life.
- SDB can cause problems at work, lost income, and mental illness.
- Untreated SDB is a major public health issue, impacting large portions of the population.

Try This

Are you tracking markers like blood pressure or blood sugar to help your doctor track your care? Start tracking your sleep as well, and see how it affects your other biomarkers.

Things to Think About

- What diseases of aging run in your family?
- How many do you already have?
- How many of your family members have been diagnosed with obstructive sleep apnea or other breathing disorders?

PART 3

Getting Help for Sleep Problems

*Our greatest weakness lies in giving up.
The most certain way to succeed is always to try
just one more time.*

—Thomas A. Edison—

If you've read this far, you may be feeling a bit worried and hopeless. After all, you've tried to get help or a good diagnosis for yourself or your child again and again. Nothing has worked before now; why should this time be any different?

I understand how hard it can be to get one wrong diagnosis after another, to be told that your problems are "resistant" to all treatment. If you've noticed yourself or your family in these pages, the reason that previous treatments haven't worked is that none of them have addressed the underlying issues.

Sleep and sleep breathing are essential to our lives. When your sleep breathing is not right, everything else falls apart. In this section, I'm going to walk you through the steps of contacting a healthcare professional, getting a screening, getting diagnosed, and finding and sticking with a treatment plan. You can do this. It won't be easy, but your life is important. Giving up and accepting the complications that come from SDB is not an option. You are important, your family and your community need you, and you can get help.

Right now, it might feel like nothing could ever make you feel better, but that's the sleepless brain talking. Let me help you get treatment, so you can be well-rested again and start living your life.

9

When You Suspect a Sleep Problem, What Comes Next?

You've read the book, you've done your research, and now you're ready to get help. But where can you go? Who can you ask for help, and what do they need to know? This chapter will explain your immediate next steps: who to talk to about screening, what information you need to bring to the screening appointment, what sort of examination they'll do, what to do if you're not taken seriously, and what sort of referrals you can expect if your care team agrees that you're at risk for SDB.

Who Can Help You Get Screened?

The first step in getting help is getting screened in a medical setting. Whether you need screening for an adult or a child, you have several options for getting help:

Your Primary Care Physician

Your PCP should be ready and willing to talk to you about sleep screenings and sleep issues. This is a common problem, and physicians working in internal medicine, family practice, and pediatrics should all have experience screening patients for sleep problems.

If you have a check-up in the near future, that can be a great time to bring up your sleep concerns. Or consider making a special appointment or messaging them through a patient portal or answering service. If you don't have a regular primary care provider or have trouble getting appointments, don't worry. Other medical providers can screen you and set you on the path to healthier sleep.

Your Dentist

Believe it or not, you can be screened for sleep issues in the dental office. Ask about the problems you've been having, and your dentist can do an oral exam to see if there are any obvious physical causes. Dentists can also refer you to specialists who can do diagnostic testing and can provide some treatments. Since many adults don't have a regular PCP but do see their dentist every six months, the dentist's office can be a great place to get screened and get referrals.

For a child, the dentist can be a great first stop since pediatric sleep apnea is often caused by issues with the tongue, palate, and jaw. Since dentists specialize in this part of the body, many pediatricians will ask for a dental evaluation as part of the diagnostic process. Dentists can also get a better look at the tonsils because our chairs are set up for reclining, and we have more tools designed for examining the mouth and throat.

Urgent Care Centers

If you don't have a relationship with a PCP or a dentist, some urgent care centers offer sleep apnea screenings and prescriptions. However, I'd also urge you to start looking for a little more stability in your care. It's helpful to have a few people who have experience caring for you and who can spot sudden changes or worrisome patterns in your health.

Specialists

If you regularly see a specialist like a cardiologist, pulmonologist, or allergist and have an appointment soon, you can ask about sleep screening and treatment. They may refer you back to your PCP for screening, but sometimes you can start the diagnosis and screening process in your specialist's office.

Emergency Room

The emergency room is generally not a good place to get treated for SDB. However, if you or someone you love is admitted to the hospital after a TIA, stroke, or heart attack, bring up a sleep screening with the doctors or nurses. SDB is a big component of these events for many people, and it could be worthwhile to be screened or diagnosed before you're sent home.

Wherever you go to get help, it's important to be clear about the symptoms, how they impact your quality of life, and what your goals are for treatment.

What Information Should You Bring to Your Sleep Screening?

For many practitioners, just being educated and concerned about the effects of sleep-disordered breathing can trigger a screening.

After all, many of us realize that this is a dangerously underrecognized problem, and we want our patients to live long, healthy lives. Professional magazines are packed with stories about how to broach the subject of SDB to patients. You *want* to have this conversation. This should be easy.

On the other hand, it's also important to keep your care team updated on what's going on with your health, what's changed, and what your specific concerns are. Remember, unless everyone you see is in the same medical organization, they may not know everything that's happened since your last appointment. And if you've been taking steps to get healthier at home, it's important to document what they were, even if they haven't been working. In fact, failed interventions can be useful information for narrowing down the sources of your issues.

When you arrive at a sleep appointment for yourself or another adult, you should have:

Home Screening Results

Screening tools can help your care team see what your concerns are and how sleep issues are affecting your daily life. Many of the standard sleep questionnaires are available online, such as the Epworth Sleepiness Scale, the STOP-BANG questionnaire, and the Pittsburgh Sleep Quality Index.

You can bring in screenshots of your results or just mention that you scored as needing to talk to a doctor on these scales. Keep in mind that your medical providers will probably want to repeat the screenings in the office, just to make sure that they have your information current.

Fitness Tracker Data

Do you wear a fitness tracker? The data can help your care team get a clearer picture of your life. How many steps do you get a day? How much exercise are you getting? What does your tracker say about your sleep, heart rate, and oxygen saturation? If you're thinking about getting a fitness tracker, you might want to get one that has good reviews for sleep tracking.

Fitness trackers can't be used for diagnostic purposes, but they're a great way to give the medical team some hard data on your life and health. It's especially important to mention if any of the data has changed since your last visit. "I used to walk 10,000 steps a day, and now I'm exhausted after 2,000" or, "My tracker says my average oxygen is below ninety at night, and it used to be about ninety-five" are important pieces of data for your doctors.

If you live alone, these trackers can be especially helpful since you don't have family members to observe your snoring, sleep breathing, or morning energy levels.

Health Data

Have you already been diagnosed with hypertension or type II diabetes? Are you tracking blood pressure or blood sugar at home? Are you an asthmatic who regularly uses a peak flow meter and tracks the data? Do you track weight? If you have numbers, and especially if you have trends or patterns, bring them with you to your sleep screening appointment. This can help pinpoint underlying issues, for instance, if your sleep is better or worse at certain times of the year. Or, if you're a woman, whether your cycles could play a role in your sleep breathing.

Snoring and Sleep Breathing Information from Family

"Do you snore?"

"Well, I don't think I do, but my wife says I snore all the time!"

This is a very common exchange in my practice. None of us like to think that we're the snorer. We always want to blame our spouse, even when we snore so loud that we wake ourselves up. If your family says you snore, ask for detailed descriptions, and take those descriptions with you to your screening. The frequency and volume of snoring can predict your risk for serious complications, so your doctor needs to know if people three rooms away are complaining or if your spouse can't sleep because of the noise.

A Complete Report of Daytime Sleepiness

Don't just say that you're kind of tired and run down. Get specific. Do you fall asleep in the dentist's chair because you can't stay awake once you stop moving? Have you fallen asleep at the wheel? Do you nod off watching TV? Let your doctor know. Believe it or not, it's not normal to be so tired that you're fighting to stay awake all the time. And, if you are falling asleep driving or operating heavy machinery, your life is in immediate danger, and your team needs to know so we can quickly get you help!

A Complete List of All Medications and Supplements You are Currently Taking

Yes, we tell you to bring this to every appointment. But that's because it's important, and it's easy to forget things in the office, especially if they're over-the-counter. Some drugs can make sleep issues worse or be deadly when combined with sleep-disordered breathing. Some supplements interact with drugs in dangerous ways. Bring the complete list.

If you want to be extra thorough, you can also mention drugs that you were prescribed but stopped taking due to side effects or because they didn't work. Sometimes, how a drug went wrong can give us hints to the underlying causes of your symptoms.

Information on Your Caffeine and Alcohol Consumption

Even if you only consume moderate amounts of caffeine and alcohol, come prepared to talk about how much you consume and when you consume them. That's because these two chemicals can have huge effects on how you sleep, how you wake, and how you feel. Plus, the amount you're drinking can be a clue to your sleep issues.

Are you drinking four huge mugs of espresso a day just to function? Do you need a glass of wine to wind down at night? These are important things to mention in a sleep screen. What you consume and when you consume it has a lot to do with what you're trying to compensate for so that you can make it through your day and your night.

Your Typical Sleep Schedule and Your Napping Habits

I'm sure your ideal sleep schedule is lovely, and in your plans, you go to bed at 9:00 every night and bounce out of bed by 6:00. We don't need to know about your ideal schedule. To help you, we need to know about your actual schedule.

Do you look at the clock at 11:00 and finally start thinking about bed?

Do you hit snooze over and over in the morning so that you're always running late?

Do you sneak in a nap after lunch, or maybe after dinner, so you can get the energy to haul the kids through their bedtime routines?

Do you find yourself wide awake at 2:00 a.m., so you have to do chores until you can fall back asleep?

This sort of data can help us figure out if your problems include circadian rhythm issues or if your sleep is so disrupted that you simply can't get enough at night.

Your Medical and Dental History

Sometimes, your dental history can give us clues about your sleep issues. Do you clench and grind your teeth? Did you have to have teeth pulled because your jaw was too small? Do you have an overbite? Did anyone ever say that you might have a tongue or lip tie? All of these issues can contribute to SDB, even in adults.

Other aspects of your medical history are also important. Did you ever have your tonsils removed? Were there any problems with your bloodwork in the past? What conditions have you been diagnosed with? Again, the more information, the easier it is to get you help quickly.

Your Family History

Sleep issues, and the problems that they cause, can run in families and cause grief generation after generation. Talk to your doctor about your entire family's health history, and especially cardiovascular issues. Make sure to mention any family history of:

- Stroke
- Arrhythmias like atrial fibrillation, long QT, palpitations
- Heart attacks
- Aneurysm
- Sudden death attributed to cardiac causes, especially during sleep

These can be signs that OSA is a family problem and that you're at high risk from untreated OSA.

Information about Your Diet

Certain food allergies, acid reflux, and diseases like alpha-gal are linked to food but can affect sleep. Come prepared to discuss when your last meal of the day is, what you tend to eat, and if you've noticed any patterns related to certain foods. For instance, if you wake up choking or gasping for breath and have stop-breathing episodes on nights that you have tomato sauce at dinner, reflux may be playing a role in your sleep breathing issues, and that's important for your doctor to know.

A List of Relevant Symptoms

Some conditions can make OSA worse or can be made worse by OSA. Be sure to mention any:

- Allergies
- Chronic nasal or sinus issues
- Morning dry mouth
- Nighttime urination
- Reflux
- Asthma
- Chronic swollen or sore throat
- Morning headaches
- Depression and anxiety
- Fatigue
- Joint pain

Giving your care team a complete list of your symptoms can help us document your need for referrals and further testing.

Your Medical Insurance Information

Since you'll probably need a referral to a specialist, your insurance information can help us connect you with a practice that is on your plan. Also, it lets us know if we need to contact the insurer when we make the referral.

If the Patient is a Child

If the patient is a child, there are a few extra pieces of useful information to bring to the screening:

- How are they doing in school? Have teachers mentioned any sleepiness? Do they get good grades and have good behavior, or do you get a lot of phone calls?
- How did they sleep as a baby? How do they sleep now? Did they have reflux or spit up a lot? Did they have trouble nursing?
- Do they wet the bed?
- Do they snore?
- How is their chewing and swallowing? Can they handle a wide range of textures? Or are they a chokey kid? Do they spit food out a lot or get it stuck in their cheeks? Are they a picky eater?
- Have they needed to see a speech and language pathologist?
- How are they at activities they enjoy? Do they have fun, or are they tired and whiney? What do their coaches and scout leaders say about them?
- What are their energy levels like at home?
- Are they a mouth breather? Do they normally hold their mouths open?
- How far can they stick out their tongue?
- How focused are they? Can they get ready to leave the house on their own? How many reminders do they need to get dressed?
- Do they have any learning, behavioral, or developmental disorders?
- Do their siblings have a history of sleep-disordered breathing?

This may seem like a lot of information to bring along to the screening appointment. Remember, several different kinds of specialists deal with sleep issues and even with sleep breathing issues. Getting a clear picture of how your sleep is affected and what your symptoms are from day to day allows us to make sure that we examine all trouble areas and make the most helpful referrals for your care.

What to Expect During a Sleep Screening Appointment

Screening appointments can vary depending on your provider, your symptoms, and your age. However, here are things that could happen during the appointment. Notice that none are particularly invasive, so there's no reason to be scared! Your care team wants to get you sleeping and breathing well so that you can live a long healthy life. They're on your side, and you don't need to feel like you're bothering them with your concerns. Your body needs to do the work of sleep, and screening is the first step towards finding out why good sleep eludes you.

Sleep Screening Questionnaires

Even if you took a screening at home, your care team will probably give you either a verbal or a written screening in the office. This is both so that they can document your sleep issues and because different offices have different preferred questionnaires.

- **The Epworth Sleepiness Scale.** This used to be the standard for diagnosing sleep disorders, and many teams still include it in the diagnostic process. It rates the severity of your sleep disorder by your reports on how likely you are to fall asleep during daily activities. One problem is this scale misses many people with SDB who are thin, young, or who have chronic illnesses that prevent activity.

In all three of these cases, the patient is often very tired but does not actually fall asleep at inappropriate times. So, while the ESS can spot the most severe cases of SDB and the people most in danger of car or workplace accidents, it misses too many other patients to be the primary tool for screening.

- **The Pittsburgh Sleep Quality Index.** The Pittsburgh index goes into more detail about specific aspects of sleep and sleep-related behaviors. It can be more useful than the ESS since it focuses on issues besides daytime sleepiness. It gives the clinician more information to start conversations with you about your sleep.

- **STOP-BANG.** The STOP-BANG scale is a simple eight-question list that is very good at detecting patients with moderate to severe obstructive sleep apnea. One problem is that it misses people in the early stages of the disease or who have UARS. However, getting treated for sleep-breathing issues early can help prevent the cardiovascular and metabolic damage that leads to full-blown OSA. So while this is a useful screening, it needs to be used in conjunction with other tools.

- **Pediatric Screening Tools.** Most pediatric sleep screening tools involve a questionnaire for parents. One problem is that many of the proven tools are aimed at children from ages six to twelve, and some of them ask about behaviors that vary by culture. However, all of them include key questions about things like daytime behavior, bedwetting, and snoring.

The Physical Exam

The sort of physical exam you'll receive depends on where you're being screened. In your primary care physician's office, you'll have your weight and blood pressure checked. Your doctor will examine your nose and throat for any obvious problems with your tongue or tonsils. If the appointment is for your child, it may be hard to get a good look at the tonsils in the general practice office, and so you'll probably have to wait for a referral to get a more complete exam.

In the dental office, the exam is a little more detailed simply because the mouth and jaw area is our specialty. That means we have the expertise and tools to get a little more information.

For instance, we'll check your palate. In a healthy mouth, the tongue rests at the top of the palate during sleep. However, if you have a high, narrow palate or a tethered tongue, your tongue rests lower in the mouth and can make it difficult to breathe in your sleep. High palates also affect the shape of your sinus cavity. This makes you more vulnerable to blockages and can lead to mouth breathing.

The teeth can also be a clue to sleep breathing issues. Many people who have SDB also clench their jaws or grind their teeth as they struggle to breathe at night. Signs of damage to your teeth can indicate a problem getting air in the night. Jaws that are too small or in the wrong position for good breathing can give you a crossbite or other tooth positioning problems. An uncorrected overbite can obstruct your sleep breathing as well. Dry mouth and untreated reflux can both cause recognizable damage to your teeth, so we may also find signs of these symptoms during the exam.

Finally, as dentists, we have the mirrors and chairs to get a good look at your tongue, throat, and tonsils to see if there are signs of swelling. In some patients with SDB, the tonsils nearly or actually touch! By examining your tongue and tonsils while you're reclined, we can get a better sense of how open your airways are when you're sleeping.

What to Do If You're Not Being Taken Seriously

Most medical providers know to be on the lookout for SDB in patients who are overweight or who have comorbidities like type II diabetes or high blood pressure. But even physicians can overlook the early stages of the disease, especially in a very high-energy child or in an adult who is thin and active. This is a huge problem since the issues related to SDB progress over time. So, while you might be thin and active now, over time, you'll gain weight, get more exhausted, and damage your cardiovascular system.

The best way to convince a provider is with hard data. Consider getting a wearable fitness monitor or pulse-oximeter and monitor your sleep for a few weeks so that you can show patterns for sleep cycles and blood oxygen levels. If your child snores and stops breathing, record them doing it, and bring the phone video in for your doctor. If your spouse has told you that you snore, have them record it. If you live alone, consider using an app to record and analyze your snoring patterns. Once you have proof that your sleep breathing is abnormal, you can return to the office and ask for more testing.

If, even with hard data, no one will take your snoring and other symptoms seriously, it may be time to make an appointment with a provider who is a member of the American Academy of Sleep Medicine, of American Academy of Dental Sleep Medicine, or who has had extra education or training in the area of sleep sciences.

Sleep medicine has made huge advances over the last two decades, so if your normal providers haven't had continuing education in the field of sleep science, they may be screening based on old stereotypes instead of the most recent data. The problem is that the old stereotypes are what happens after years of neglected SDB. The most recent data suggests that we can prevent serious complications, and even sudden death, by being proactive about screening and treatment. **You deserve to be taken seriously**. Professionals who have made an effort to stay up-to-date on sleep medicine will help you.

What Kinds of Referrals Will I Get?

Who you or your child is referred to varies depending on what underlying problems could be causing the SDB. Common referrals can include:

WHEN YOU SUSPECT A SLEEP PROBLEM, WHAT COMES NEXT?

- An ear, nose, and throat specialist to see if you have physical problems that prevent nasal breathing
- A dentist, orthodontist, or oral surgeon if there are issues involving tongue and lip ties, the palate, or the jaw
- A speech and language pathologist, occupational therapist, or oral myofunctional therapist for issues with muscle tone and tongue movement
- A sleep lab for an overnight sleep study
- A cardiologist to rule out any heart defects or arrhythmias
- A pulmonologist if lung problems are suspected
- An allergist if your sleep breathing issues could be caused by asthma or allergies
- Bloodwork to eliminate other causes for your symptoms

Sometimes, you might receive more than one referral as part of exploring the next steps for you or your loved one. It can be intimidating, but remember, the goal is to find underlying causes and treat them so that you can live a long and healthy life. These next appointments are all part of the diagnostic process. In the next chapter, I'll explain some of the tests and appointments that will contribute to your diagnosis. Unknown things are scary, but if you read on, you'll see that these routine diagnostic tests are safe and full of great information for you and your care team.

The Take-Aways

- A dentist, physician, specialist, or even an urgent care center can screen you for sleep issues and get you started on the road to better sleep.
- Home fitness trackers and online sleep assessments can help you see if you have a sleeping problem.

- If one provider won't take your sleep concerns seriously, get a second opinion. Your health matters!

Try This

If you suspect that you have sleep issues and haven't made a screening appointment yet, do it now. Put down the book, pick up the phone, and make that appointment.

Things to Think About

- Has your sleep quality gotten worse over the last few years?
- Have you tried to track sleep with a fitness tracker? What did it tell you?
- Which provider will you talk to about sleep?

10

What Do All These Tests Mean and Will They Hurt?

Getting medical tests can be pretty scary. But the tests to diagnose your sleep and breathing issues aren't dangerous, and most of them aren't even a tiny bit painful. It's easy to put off a diagnosis because you feel like you don't have time or that other things are more important. But remember, every day you go without healthy, healing sleep, you're doing damage to your mind and body. Get diagnosed and treated now so you can prevent permanent health problems.

Polysomnography: Everything You Ever Wanted to Know About Lab-Based Sleep Studies

The words "sleep lab" sound intimidating. Labs are usually places where we get poked with needles. People do experiments in labs. And now your care team has asked you to spend all night in one? How can they expect you to sleep at all in such a scary place?

Sleep labs do not involve needles.

That's right. No needles. And the only "experiment" they'll be doing is using sensors to record what happens to your brain and body while you sleep. Sleep labs can be at hospitals or free-standing sleep centers. Your room is a bedroom with a private bathroom that looks a bit like a hotel room. It's designed to help you be comfortable so that you can get a good night's sleep.

Different centers have different standards for sleep study start and end times. If you usually stay up very late, or if you're a shift worker, tell them when you book your appointment. The sleep study team wants the study to coincide with your sleepiest time of the day or night. That will help them get at least four to six hours of good sleep data for you.

For most adult sleep studies, you cannot have a support person in the room with you during the night. However, if you have special needs and require extra support, let the sleep center know. You should also let them know if you have any health conditions that could require extra monitoring overnight.

The sleep center will give you a list of instructions for the day before your appointment. Most will tell you to avoid alcohol on the day of your study and to stop drinking caffeine after noon. You should eat dinner before you go to the sleep lab for the evening. Some labs ask that you shower before you arrive. **Do not nap on the day of a sleep study.**

When you pack for your night in the sleep center, pack as if you're going to a hotel overnight. Bring:

- Toothbrush and toothpaste
- Haircare items

- Washcloth, towel, and your favorite soap
- Phone or music device
- White noise device if you use one
- Loose-fitting pajamas
- Clothes for the next day
- Medications and sanitary products
- Evening and morning snacks
- Book, knitting, or another typical evening quiet activity
- Slippers or socks

When you get to the sleep center, you'll change into a pair of your own comfortable pajamas. Choose a loose-fitting pair so that it will work with the monitoring equipment. You must wear pajamas at the sleep center, even if you sleep without them at home. The temperature in the room will be adjusted so that you're comfortable in your pajamas.

You can have a bedtime snack, brush your teeth, and take your medicines just like at home. The sleep study team will attach about twenty different sensors to your scalp, temples, chest, and legs with a mild adhesive. These don't hurt, but they'll measure what your brain, heart, lungs, and muscles are doing while you sleep. Many centers have televisions in the rooms, most have Wi-Fi, and you can always bring a book or puzzle. The team wants you to be comfortable so you can fall and stay asleep.

After you fall asleep, the sensors will record the stage of sleep that you're in, your blood oxygen levels, and if you have any unusual brain, muscles, or breathing patterns while you sleep. If your apnea is very obvious, the team may wake you up and give you a machine to help you breathe for the second half of the night to record the difference with and without breathing help.

The sleep team is in the next room all night, so if you need to get up and use the restroom, need a drink, or need some other kind of help, you can call them. In the morning, when you get up, they'll remove the sensors, you can take any medications, and eat a snack if you've brought one. Some centers have showers; at others, you'll have to go home to shower.

Sleep studies usually end by 7:00 a.m. but may end earlier or later, depending on the sleep center. After the study is complete, you'll need to have an appointment with your physician to discuss your results and plan further tests or your treatment.

How Sleep Studies Differ for Children

If you're taking a child to a sleep study, there are a few major differences:

- Sleep studies for children often start earlier since children go to bed earlier and need more sleep.
- A parent or guardian can remain in the room all night. At some centers, they're required to remain in the room.
- Sleep studies for children need to be conducted at a center that is qualified to study pediatric patients. That way, they have the proper equipment on hand and technicians who can deal with children. If possible, have a pediatric study done at a center associated with a children's hospital. Children's hospitals are experts at helping kids feel comfortable and calm during tests and medical procedures.
- In addition to the other items, pack their favorite stuffed toy, bedtime stories, or DVDs. The goal is to mimic their bedtime routine as closely as possible and to help them fall asleep quickly.

Home Studies

If you are an adult who can't have a study in a sleep lab, a home sleep study can be an alternative diagnostic tool. In a home study, you wear fewer sensors, set up the equipment yourself, and sleep in your own bed. Homes studies are much less expensive than overnight studies at a sleep lab.

Home studies are limited in their diagnostic capabilities. They can diagnose OSA, but they can't rule out a diagnosis of OSA. Some newer units even track microarousals and stages of sleep. They cannot be used with children. However, if you have the symptoms of OSA and many of the risk factors for it, you may be able to use a home sleep study kit instead of spending a night at a sleep lab.

What are Sleep Studies Looking For?

When your care team looks at your study results, they'll be paying close attention to a few different numbers.

They'll look at the apnea-hypopnea index (AHI). This is the average number of times in an hour that your airway is partially or totally blocked. An AHI greater than or equal to five in an adult or greater than or equal to one in a child means that you have diagnosable OSA and need treatment.

Using AHI alone identifies the most severe cases of sleep breathing, so the sleep lab will also use the Respiratory Disturbance Index (RDI). This number also includes microarousals where the patient is struggling to breathe but where the airflow hasn't yet been severely blocked. For instance, if someone wakes up, adjusts their position, and goes back to sleep, that's included in the RDI. Using the RDI allows the team to identify people who are missing out on the work of sleep and who may progress to full-blown OSA if they don't receive treatment soon.

The sleep study will also give your team data on how your blood oxygen changes during sleep. In a healthy sleeper, oxygen saturation remains above 95% all night long. People with mild SDB see their sats dip as low as 86%. If someone's sats fall below 79%, they have severe sleep breathing issues.

Finally, your team will look at the time you spend in each sleep stage, if your muscles moved oddly during sleep, and if you appear to have any heart problems. After all, some people have more than one sleep problem at a time, and your team will want to address all of them.

A good practitioner of sleep medicine will take your numbers as part of the story but also take into account the impact that poor sleep quality is having on your daily life. Someone with an AHI of five who routinely falls asleep at the wheel is in more immediate danger than someone with an AHI of fifteen who feels mostly fine all day long.

Why Do I Need to See An Allergist?

If your care team suspects that your issues with SDB may be due to problems with nasal breathing, they may send you to see an allergist. Nearly half of all Americans have at least one allergy, and both food and environmental allergies can affect your breathing. The allergist will ask you about your symptoms and then do skin tests and blood tests.

Both of these do involve needles and some discomfort. For the blood test, the allergist will draw blood and send it to a lab to identify potential allergens. In the skin test, the allergist uses a tool that lets him scratch your skin, usually on your back, with up to 50 common allergens at once. The size of your skin's reaction to the allergen will tell him how allergic you are to each one. While the scratches themselves don't hurt, it can be painful if you turn out to be severely allergic to one of the items on the test.

You'll be able to get immediate feedback on if you have allergies, what they are, medications to take, and how to eliminate allergens from your sleeping area. Many patients are shocked at how quickly their sleep quality and sleep breathing improves once they put all of the allergist's recommendations in place.

Mira had always snored and breathed through her mouth at night, but I didn't want to explore options like surgery until we'd seen if there were other ways to fix her breathing. When we went to the allergist, we found out that she was extremely reactive to dust and mold. We live in a humid climate, so mold is a year-round problem, and the allergist explained that no matter how clean you keep your home, there will be dust. We replaced her carpet with laminate, started washing her bedding on hot, got dust covers, and put a HEPA filter in her room. We also started her on some OTC allergy meds recommended by her allergist.

When we went back to her pediatrician a month later, it was like we had brought him a totally different kid. Her throat looked great, she was breathing through her nose, and her skin had cleared up too. I feel like we were lucky to have such a simple fix. It had never occurred to us that her bedroom was keeping her from sleeping and breathing well.

—Mother of Mira (9)—

Bloodwork for Better Sleep

Could the reason you're so tired be in your blood? It's a good idea to get bloodwork done as part of the diagnostic process. If you have

OSA and another health problem as well, the treatments for OSA will be more successful and give you faster results if you also take care of any other systemic issues.

Your physician may want to check and make sure that:

- Your vitamins D, B12, B6, and iron levels are high enough
- Your blood counts are correct
- You don't have an existing infection that your body is trying to fight off
- Your thyroid is working properly
- You don't have celiac disease
- Your blood sugar is in range, both when you fast and over the long term (with your a1c levels)

If you haven't had a blood test in a while, they can be scary, but you don't have to watch, and if you're afraid of fainting, you can ask the lab to take your blood lying down. Getting blood tests is especially important if you experience dangerous levels of daytime sleepiness. Many disorders can cause that, and your doctor wants you to be in the best health possible.

What the ENT Can Tell You about Your Sleep Breathing

For children, the ENT is often the next stop after a sleep screen detects issues. This is because the most common cause of SDB in children is enlarged tonsils and adenoids. The ENT is the specialist who can perform a tonsillectomy and adenectomy, usually the first line of treatment for kids with sleep breathing problems.

However, some adults also benefit from seeing an ENT. If you have loud snoring or impaired nasal breathing, you may have underlying physical issues in your nose or sinuses. The ENT can examine you to spot underlying problems causing SDB. Fixing these problems can make your SDB treatments more effective.

The ENT will perform a physical exam with a light. If she decides she needs a better view of your nose, sinuses, and throat, she may also use a fiberoptic tube with a camera and light. This doesn't hurt, but it may feel uncomfortable or make you gag. However, ENTs have a lot of practice with this tool, and it will just be a quick look.

If the ENT suspects you may have sinus polyps or some other serious issue contributing to your sleep breathing problems, she may also recommend a CT scan of your sinuses. CT scans don't hurt, and the scanner is shaped like a donut—you're not in an enclosed space. The images from the scan will help the ENT determine whether your OSA treatment plan needs to include sinus or nasal surgery.

Cardiologists to Rule Out Heart Issues

If your care team suspects that heart issues may be contributing to your daytime sleepiness or sleep problems, they may refer you to a cardiologist. A cardiologist will usually ask for an echocardiogram. An echocardiogram is basically an ultrasound but of a heart. The technician will move the wand around and ask you to breathe, hold your breath, or change position at certain points. The echo can show the team how blood is moving through your heart, if there are any physical abnormalities, and if you have irregular heart rhythms during the test.

Echocardiograms do not hurt, and you lie on a bed during them. After the test, the cardiologist interprets the images and either meets with you or sends a report to the referring doctor. If you have heart irregularities contributing to sleep breathing issues, they can often be treated with medications that improve heart function or reduce the amount of work your heart has to do.

Pulmonologist to Rule Out Lung Issues

Your care team may refer you to the pulmonologist if they suspect that your SDB may be made worse by general breathing issues. If someone has asthma or COPD, they don't breathe well day or night, especially when they're lying down. They may struggle to breathe at night and wake frequently. For instance, if you have a child with asthma, you've probably lain awake at night listening to their nagging cough. Adults with asthma have similar issues, but often there's no one to alert them or their physicians to the night coughing.

The pulmonologist will do lung function tests to see if your lungs and the airways in your chest are working properly. You'll have to breathe deeply and exhale at different rates so they can measure things like:

- Lung capacity
- How quickly and powerfully you can exhale
- If you can efficiently empty your lungs
- If you can breathe in without struggling

If you have a lung or airway condition in addition to SDB, the pulmonologist can prescribe medications or exercises to improve your lungs and improve your breathing during the day and at night.

Dentists to Fix Mouth and Palate Issues

If your screening wasn't done at the dental office and your care team wants to rule out oral abnormalities that contribute to SDB, you'll be referred to a dentist. The tests at the dentist will probably include a full oral exam and possibly x-rays.

Your dentist will ask you to move your tongue around, will check the shape of your palate, look for signs of an overbite, and check your molars for signs of grinding or clenching. This exam is quick and painless. It does not include any scraping, needles, or drills.

Why Would I Need to See a Therapist?

You may need to have an evaluation with a speech, occupational, or oral myofunctional therapist as part of your diagnostic process. These experts can diagnose problems with your tongue, mouth, and throat muscles that may be causing sleep-disordered breathing.

For your evaluation, you'll be asked to move in certain ways, make certain sounds, and perhaps even chew and swallow. Often, people have been living with disorders that they've worked around for years. These therapists can determine if any of the issues causing SDB are treatable with special exercises. For instance, they can help someone learn to use nasal rather than oral breathing patterns or to rest their tongue on the roof of the mouth rather than the floor of the mouth.

Starting the Process

The diagnostic process for SDB includes finding and treating underlying conditions, but as you can see, most of these tests aren't painful. It's important to make appointments and follow through with your care team's suggestions. You want the best possible, personalized treatment that will give you productive, efficient sleep and prevent future disease.

The Take-Aways

- Sleep studies do not hurt.
- You may have to see one or more specialists to rule out underlying conditions.
- It is worth taking the necessary time to improve your sleep.

Try This

If you think you may need referrals to specialists, check to see who's on your insurance before you go in for your screening appointment. That will help speed the process up.

Things to Think About

- What do you need to do a sleep study? Do you need transportation? Childcare?
- Would an at-home sleep study be a better fit for your life?

… 11

How We Fix Broken Sleep

This book is ultimately about good news. Bad sleep and bad sleep breathing have terrible consequences. If you get screened, diagnosed, and treated, you can avoid those consequences. Sometimes, if we catch your issues early enough, we can even reverse the damage that's already happened. With treatments like the ones in this chapter, we can give you your life back. If you, a partner, or a child have signs of SDB, these are the treatments that can help. Different people benefit from different types of treatment, and not everyone tolerates every treatment. But don't give up. Communicate with your care team. If you don't seem to be getting results from your current treatment plan, ask about your other options.

Learn to Love Your Circadian Rhythms

One of the easiest ways to fix your sleep is to get to know your circadian rhythms and adjust your schedule to suit them. Go off alcohol and after-lunch caffeine for a few days, and pay attention to your body. When do you naturally want to fall asleep? When there's no alarm, when do you wake up? Many people who have sleep problems actually have schedule problems.

Do you wake up every day at four in the morning, unable to get back to sleep? Try going to sleep by eight so you can get a full night of rest. Maybe you or your teen is a night owl who isn't sleepy before midnight? See how much you can adjust your schedule to let you wake up later. (Night owls have it harder than extreme morning people because our society prizes an early start.) If you can't get your circadian rhythm to match with your job, school, or family life, talk to a physician. But keep in mind that it's difficult to shift our body clocks—they're controlled by genes—so you may have better luck trying to find work or class schedules that fit with your natural tendencies.

Can Cognitive Therapy Help You Sleep Better?

Cognitive behavioral therapy (CBT) is a therapy designed to break bad thought patterns and teach people healthier ways to think and behave. It can build better habits and give patients a toolbox of coping strategies to use in tough situations.

CBT has long been used for disorders like anxiety, depression, and addiction. Marriage counselors sometimes use it to help couples break out of bad patterns. However, in recent years, sleep scientists have realized that it can also be helpful for treating sleeping difficulties.

Insomnia

For someone with insomnia, it can be difficult to get to sleep or stay asleep. Over time, the sleeper's relationship with sleep becomes stressful. Sleep becomes so worrisome that worries about sleep keep the patient awake. CBT for insomnia is aimed at teaching the patient the skills involved in getting a good night's sleep. The course of therapy and the therapy homework is often personalized for the patient but usually includes:

- Good sleep hygiene and how to prepare the body and mind for sleep
- How to avoid lying awake in bed
- What to do after a night-waking
- Daytime habits to encourage night-time sleepiness
- Relaxation and mediation tricks
- Avoiding bad narratives about sleep and wakefulness
- Changing your "head voice" to avoid sleep worry
- Biofeedback to learn what "sleepiness" feels like

With CBT, patients with insomnia often learn how to fall asleep and to stay asleep all night.

SDB and Insomnia

SDB can often lead to insomnia. Over time, the stress of sleep convinces the brain that sleep isn't safe. Patients develop anxiety related to falling asleep, and they may get up after a RERA and stay up. For patients with SDB and insomnia, simply treating one of the conditions isn't enough. SDB treatments can't work if the patient isn't actually sleeping. Improving insomnia alone can't fix the problems with sleep because the brain and body still aren't getting adequate oxygen.

However, for these patients, a combination of SDB treatments and CBT can yield big improvements. CBT helps the patients get to sleep, stay asleep, and comply with treatment plans. The SDB treatments improve breathing. The combination results in a good night's sleep.

SDB Alone

CBT has also been shown to improve outcomes in patients with SDB but not insomnia. That's because the CBT gives them the tools they need to adhere to treatment plans, make changes in their sleeping environment, and engage in healthy daytime behaviors that support sleep breathing. CBT can give patients the confidence, problem-solving skills, and practice they need to ensure their SDB treatment is a success.

Where to Get CBT for Sleep-Related Issues

CBT can be in person, but it doesn't have to be. You can get effective sleep-related SDB from:

- A local independent practitioner
- A hospital or sleep center
- By telemedicine
- Through certain smartphone apps like the free *Insomnia Coach* app developed by the Veterans Administration

You don't have to fix your sleep habits on your own. Getting help means that you'll be healthier and live longer.

Oral-Myofunctional Therapy to Aid in the Work of Sleep

An oral myofunctional therapist specializes in training the muscles of the throat, tongue, and mouth to work together. Since muscle weakness and lack of tone can contribute to UARS and SDB, working with a therapist can help you reduce snoring, AHIs, and microarousals. Some areas where an OMT can help are:

- Tongue control and tone
- Proper tongue placement during sleep

- Lower jaw strength and positioning
- Throat muscles
- Soft palate stiffness
- Encouraging nasal breathing

You can find OMTs associated with occupational and physical therapy groups, speech and language pathology groups, and dental offices. Ask your care team if an OMT could help you learn to reduce snoring and AHIs.

Why Do People Keep Mentioning Melatonin?

Melatonin is the hormone that helps us go to sleep and stay asleep. Some people find that it helps them deal with sleep issues related to anxiety, ASD, insomnia, shiftwork, or circadian rhythms.

In recent years, melatonin has become very popular among parents as a safe sleep aid for children. Many adults also take melatonin supplements to help them get to sleep.

In general, doctors recommend improving sleep hygiene and getting CBT before trying supplements or medications to aid sleep. However, if you've tried these interventions for yourself or your child, your physician may recommend trying melatonin supplements to see if they work for you.

Melatonin supplements vary from manufacturer to manufacturer and batch to batch. If a medical provider recommends them to you, be sure to ask for information on which supplements to buy and how to dose them.

Changing Your Sleeping Environment for Better Sleep

Sometimes, all it takes to sleep better and to heal your airway is a better sleeping environment. By making changes in your sleeping environment, you can alleviate some of the underlying conditions that lead to insomnia, UARS, or mild SDB.

Get a Healthy Bedtime Routine

A healthy bedtime routine can promote good sleep and sleep breathing:

- Avoid eating too close to bedtime.
- Take a hot shower to remove allergens from your body and to help lower your core temperature.
- Don't have caffeine and alcohol before bed.
- Don't get into bed until you're ready to wind down for sleep.

Keep Screens out of the Bedroom

I know; your phone is like a part of your body. You check it first thing in the morning and last thing before bed. The problem is, the blue light from electronics like phones, computers, tablets, and televisions can mess with your melatonin production and your circadian rhythm. Try to cut off screens and blue light from LED bulbs at least an hour or two before bed. If you can't go cold turkey, switch to baby steps. Try reading, knitting, sketching, or listening to music or books to help you wind down to sleep. If you prefer e-books to physical copies, put the phone or tablet away and reach for an e-ink reader instead. Your brain will sleep better, and you'll wake better.

Sleep Cold

Did you know researchers have found the ideal bedroom temperature to promote deep, restful sleep? If you're like most Americans, your bedroom is probably a touch too warm. Set your thermostat to 65 degrees, and you'll sleep longer, better, and more deeply.

Think About Your Window Treatments

It can be nice to wake up to morning light, but the way that daylight varies over the year can really do a number on your sleep. Consider getting room-darkening curtains or shades so that you can have darkness when you need to sleep.

White Noise or Noise Cancelling—The Choice is Yours

If your sleep is frequently interrupted by things that go bump in the night or zoom down the highway and you don't need to parent small children, consider getting either a white noise generator or noise-canceling headphones. Try both and see what works best for you. Some people find white noise aggravating; others are made anxious by noise cancellation technology. The key is to make your room a safe, calm place that supports the work of sleep.

Humidifiers, Especially in the Winter

Dry air is hard on your airways. Your nose is supposed to humidify the air before it reaches your lungs, but if the air in your bedroom is too dry, the lining of your nose and sinuses can swell or even bleed. This will cause more breathing effort. You'll either wake up repeatedly all night or start mouth breathing, irritating your throat and airways. A humidifier can make the air in your room easier to breathe and soothe your nose.

Air Filters

Air filters like HEPA filters or ionic filters can remove particles from the air. Even if you don't have environmental allergies, excessive dust, pet dander, mold spores, pollen, or pollution can irritate your airways and make it harder to breathe. Air filters can be a cost-effective way to reduce the effects of UARS so that you can get more uninterrupted sleep.

Sleeping Position

For mild UARS, how you sleep can affect how you breathe. Sleeping on your side or sleeping in an elevated position may help you breathe better. Special pillows designed to support a better sleeping position may help you breathe so that your body can do the work of sleep.

Allergy Treatments Can Improve Sleep Outcomes

If your allergy appointment resulted in a diagnosis, your sleep disorder treatment plan will include treating your allergies. There are many safe and effective ways to treat allergies to improve sleep.

Change Your Sleeping Space

One of the first-line SDB treatments for people whose allergies include substances like dust, mold, and pet dander is to allergy-proof your sleeping space. We're in our bedrooms for eight hours straight, and when they're full of allergens, we can't breathe well. Common ways to reduce allergens in the bedroom are:

- Using a HEPA filter at night
- Dust-proof mattress and pillow covers
- Keeping dirty laundry out of the bedroom and off the floor

- Replacing carpets with hardwood, laminate, or tile flooring. If your feet get cold, use washable throw rugs or slippers.
- Banning pets (real or stuffed) from the bed
- Showering before bed to remove allergens from skin and hair
- Washing all bedding on hot once a week

The fewer allergens that you allow into your bedroom, the easier it will be to sleep and breathe.

Over-the-Counter Allergy Pills

Many allergy pills can be used long-term, control symptoms well, and are safe with very few side effects. Cetirizine, loratadine, and fexofenadine are all inexpensive and available at most stores. Different people prefer different pills. Ask your allergist for suggestions on which pill to choose and what dose to take.

Over-the-Counter Nose Sprays

Nose sprays like Fluticasone are more expensive per-dose than allergy pills, but if your nose and sinuses are interfering with your sleep breathing, they're an excellent treatment option. In many cases, the right combination of OTC sprays and pills can improve or even cure snoring and improve daytime sleepiness and sleep quality.

Once-A-Day Maintenance Inhalers

If your allergies cause your airways to swell and make it harder to breathe, the allergist may prescribe a steroid inhaler to control your symptoms. These are usually once-a-day medications and are safe to take long term. The one drawback is that if your insurance has a high deductible or high drug copays, these inhalers can be very expensive.

Rescue Inhalers

If your sleep is frequently interrupted by a nagging dry cough caused by allergens, the allergist may also prescribe an albuterol rescue inhaler. However, if you're using this more than occasionally, talk to your medical team. They'll want to adjust your other medicines.

Allergy Shots

Finally, if allergies severely impact your sleep breathing and can't be cured with other interventions, your allergist may recommend three to five years of allergy shots. Allergy shots introduce small amounts of an allergen into your body. Over time, your immune system stops reacting to the allergen, and your allergic reaction improves. Allergy shots are expensive, and so most insurers will only cover them if other treatments have failed.

PAP Machines: Why Do I Need One and Why Are There So Many Types?

If you complete an at-home or in-lab sleep study, your care team will probably prescribe you a PAP machine. A PAP is a positive airway pressure machine. To use a PAP machine, you wear a mask when you go to sleep. The machine forces a constant stream of air through your nose and throat. This keeps your airways open so you can breathe easily and without obstruction. A properly worn PAP will reduce or eliminate apneas, hypopneas, and RERAs so that your sleep is less interrupted and you can get better rest.

A CPAP, a continuous positive airway pressure machine, is often the first machine that a physician will recommend, though the automatic positive airway pressure machine is becoming more popular. The third kind of machine is called a BiPAP. It alternates between two pressure settings and is sometimes used for patients with specific objections to the CPAP.

CPAP DIAGRAM

Nasal Mask

Obstructive Apnea/Hypopnea

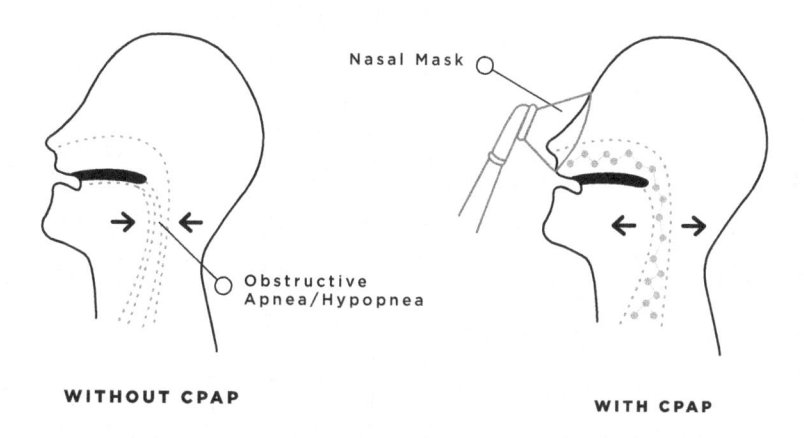

WITHOUT CPAP

WITH CPAP

Figure 9. The pressure from the airflow of a PAP machine holds the airway open so that the body can get enough oxygen at night.

CPAP Therapy

The CPAP provides a single level of air pressure to your nose and throat. The mask can cover just your nose, or both your nose and mouth. Most CPAPs also contain a humidifier so that the air will be easier to breathe. The pressure for your CPAP is often set during your sleep study and needs to be checked and adjusted by your doctor.

CPAPs have been in use for over thirty years and are well-studied. They can cause problems in people who have difficulty getting their mask to fit correctly, who change position frequently while sleeping, and who are prone to ear and sinus infections.

CPAP pressure is based in part on your weight, so if you gain or lose more than 10% of your body weight, the pressure needs to be readjusted. Otherwise, you can get ear infections, or swallow air and have painful gas. Some patients also panic when exhaling and fight the CPAP. Many modern CPAPs have a setting called "expiration pressure release," which can help with this feeling. Physicians can also refer you to CBT if your CPAP causes anxiety.

APAP Therapy

Some patients prefer APAP therapy to CPAP therapy. Many insurance plans do not differentiate between APAP and CPAP machines. APAP machines don't require a sleep lab to adjust the pressure. APAP machines adjust their pressure automatically in response to your body's needs. This includes adjusting for weight, sleeping position, and stage of sleep.

APAPs are more expensive than CPAPs and can't be used by people with heart failure. However, they're a good option for people who need more flexibility in the amount of airflow at night.

BiPAP Therapy

BiPAP therapy can sometimes be helpful for people who find the CPAP's pressure unbearable. BIPAPs use higher pressure when you inhale and a lower pressure when you exhale. They're better than the CPAP for patients who don't breathe enough, for people who swallow air on the CPAP, or for people who find the CPAP claustrophobic and panic-inducing. Because they are very expensive, insurers will generally not cover them until a patient has failed at using a CPAP or APAP.

PAP Therapy and Children

PAP therapy is not the first line of treatment for children but may be prescribed if a child still has symptoms of OSA after surgery. Children often have trouble complying with these machines because they are uncomfortable, it's hard to get a good mask fit, and growth spurts can lead to frequent adjustments. If your pediatrician has suggested you try a PAP machine and it's not working for your child, ask about other treatments.

CPAP Machine Care

It's important to clean your machine and replace parts as directed. If you allow the machine to get dirty, you'll put yourself at risk for skin, lung, ear, and sinus infections.

- Wash the mask, tubes, and water chamber daily.
- Wash the headgear and filter weekly.
- Soak the water chamber in vinegar weekly.
- Change the disposable filter monthly.

If you care for your machine well, you'll improve your health, and it will last longer.

What if the CPAP Doesn't Work for Me?

If the CPAP doesn't work for you, and you've tried other PAP alternatives, don't give up hope! There are other non-invasive solutions for SDB. If your SDB is very severe and you've exhausted non-invasive options, you may also be a candidate for some of the invasive treatment options that I'll discuss later in the chapter.

Addressing GERD

Gastrointestinal reflux disease (GERD) can contribute to UARS. That's because the acid reflux from GERD can damage the lining of your throat and sinuses. The microarousals of UARS can also make GERD worse, so you can get into a feedback loop where both conditions are aggravating each other.

If you ever wake up with a burning, choking sensation, talk to your doctor about GERD. A physician can often spot the damage the acid has done to your throat, while your dentist can see acid damage on the teeth. Medication, dietary changes, sleeping position changes, and changes to your daily routine can all improve reflux and, as your body heals, sleep breathing.

Oral Appliance (OA) Therapy for SDB

Oral appliances can be used to treat SDB. They're recommended for adults with mild to moderate SDB or for people who can't tolerate PAP therapy. There are two common types of oral appliances for adults.

Removable Appliances

Removable appliances are designed to be worn during sleep, much like the retainers you or your friends might have had as children and teens. Before you go to bed, you place the appliance in your mouth. It adjusts your jaw position so that it's slightly forward while you sleep. This prevents your jaw and tongue from falling back and obstructing the airway. Your airway stays open all night, and you can breathe and sleep.

There are low-cost oral appliances available over the counter, but they can cause tooth or jaw issues if you use one long term. Ideally, you should use a well-fitted sleep breathing appliance from a dentist.

Your provider will take molds or images of your teeth to help in designing the oral appliance. These images are sent to a lab that will construct an appliance that fits your mouth. When it comes in, you'll need a second appointment to pick up your appliance and check the fit. After that, you will need follow up appointments and sleep studies to make sure the position of the appliance is helping keep the airway open.

In studies, these appliances have performed about as well as throat, palate, and tongue surgery, and in some cases, as well as a PAP machine. However, many patients will wear an appliance but won't use their CPAP, and a treatment plan you can follow is always better than the one you abandon. Convenience is a huge benefit of OAs for SDB:

- You can change your position easily.
- You don't need a plug or bedside table to use one.
- They fit into a pocket or a purse for easy travel.
- They don't make noise.
- They're easy to clean.
- They still work if you lose weight.
- They're a good option for people who get sinus, ear, or skin infections on PAP therapy.

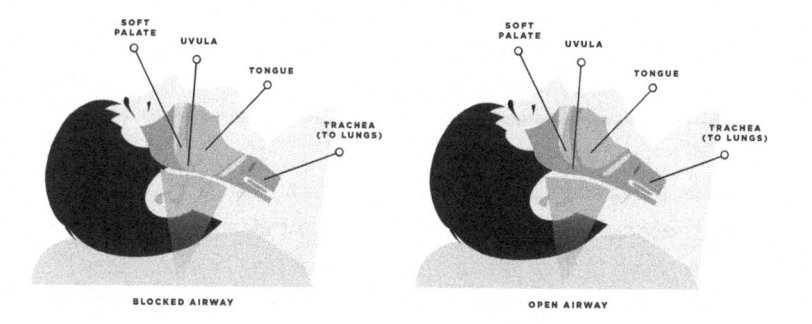

Figure 10. On the left, you can see the blocked airway of a person with OSA. On the right, an oral appliance has repositioned the tongue and jaw. This keeps the airway open at night and allows good sleep breathing.

Implanted Appliances

A newer form of appliance for OSA is a palate implant. The implant consists of three polyester rods that your ENT implants into your palate with local anesthesia. As the tissue around them heals, it stiffens and restores the function of the soft palate. This procedure can help people with UARS or mild OSA who can't tolerate PAP therapy.

Some people still need PAP therapy even after the rods are implanted, and as you age or gain weight, the therapy may become less effective. However, it may help prevent UARS from either progressing to OSA or causing damage to your arteries, and it can help you get more hours of healthy sleep each night.

Removing Tonsils and Adenoids

For children, the first line of treatment for OSA is often to remove the tonsils and adenoids. These glands react to respiratory infections and can become permanently swollen or inflamed. They can also get irritated as a result of mouth breathing, and some children just have unusually large tonsils and adenoids in an unusually small throat. Removing the glands opens the airway and can restore proper sleep breathing in children who don't have other underlying issues.

When the pediatrician talked to Corrie after her surgery, she was most excited about the slumber parties. At eleven, Corrie had never gotten to sleep over at a friend's house. Her OSA had caused bedwetting, and she didn't want to have to explain her pull-ups to the other girls in her class. Even worse, she snored. "So loudly the house seems to shake," her mother had said at the screening appointment.

Poor Corrie knew she'd be an outcast if she ever stayed the night for a party. So, instead, she told people that her mother wouldn't let her go to slumber parties. It was better to be the kid with the super-strict parents than the kid who snored and wet herself.

Within weeks of the surgery, the bedwetting and the snoring cleared up. The next time a friend had a slumber party, Corrie went and stayed all night. Her parents might be happiest about the better grades and better behavior, but for Corrie, the best part of treating her OSA was that she could finally be a normal kid who did normal kid things.

T&A DIAGRAM
FOR SURGERY

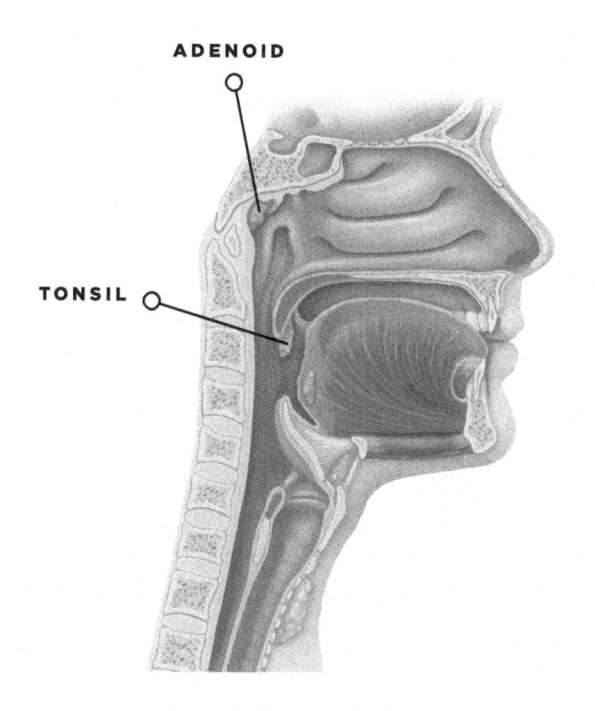

ADENOID

TONSIL

Figure 11. T&A surgery removes the tonsils and adenoids. A first-line OSA treatment for children, it is an outpatient surgery.

The surgery to remove tonsils and adenoids is an outpatient surgery. Your child will receive general anesthesia and be asleep for the procedure. After the anesthesia wears off, you can go home with ibuprofen and acetaminophen for pain management. Your child will need rest and bland, soft foods for several days, but after the surgery, sleep breathing should be improved.

For some children, T&A surgery is not enough to cure sleep breathing issues. These kids may also need other interventions to address the underlying conditions that are keeping them from breathing well.

Some adults also have chronically swollen, inflamed tonsils contributing to their sleep breathing problems, though this condition is rarer. A T&A for an adult is similar to one for a child. However, while children usually recover in seven to ten days after surgery, adults often take a full fourteen days to recover.

Surgeries of Last Resort

If you're unable to tolerate any of the non-invasive methods for dealing with SDB, there are inpatient surgeries that can open your airway and treat your SDB. However, the American Academy of Sleep Medicine emphasizes that surgery is irreversible, often dangerous, and not always guaranteed to provide a lasting cure, especially as people age or gain weight.

UPPP and UPPGP

Uvulopalatopharyngoplasty (UPPP) and Uvulopalatopharyngoglossoplasty (UPPGP) are surgeries that open the airway by removing the excess tissue from the:

- uvula
- tonsils

- adenoids
- soft palate
- throat
- and tongue

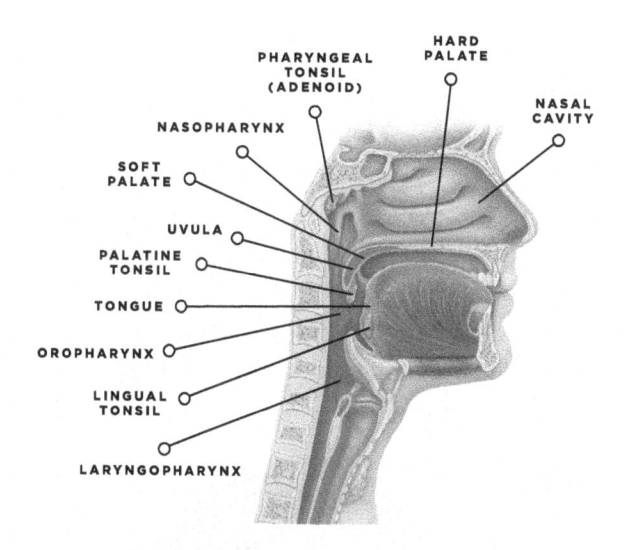

Figure 12. Since UPPGP surgery tackles multiple potential blockages at once, it can be hard to recover from.

This surgery is best for people with mild to moderate OSA who have been unable to benefit from PAP devices and who have physical abnormalities of these tissues. However, even with these caveats, this inpatient surgery only benefits about 40% of patients. It takes two to three weeks to make a full recovery, and even those patients who see a cure may develop OSA again later or still need a PAP machine after therapy.

Mandibular Maxillary Advancement

Mandibular Maxillary Advancement surgery requires an overnight stay in the ICU and two to three days inpatient, as well as several weeks of recovery. In this surgery, the upper and lower jaw and muscles are repositioned to eliminate the airway obstruction. About 50% of the patients who undergo this surgery will see their sleep apnea cured, and 95% of patients say that their face looks the same or better after the surgery. This surgery can help people, even obese people, with moderate to severe OSA who can't tolerate PAP therapy.

Tracheostomy

This is the last resort for OSA surgery because it is disfiguring, can affect speech and social life, and can lead to reoccurring, serious airway infections. In a tracheostomy, a hole is made in the windpipe below the upper airway. Patients bypass the upper airway when breathing at night, and so they no longer have apneas. While this is a serious operation, it can save the lives of patients when all other non-invasive and surgical interventions have failed.

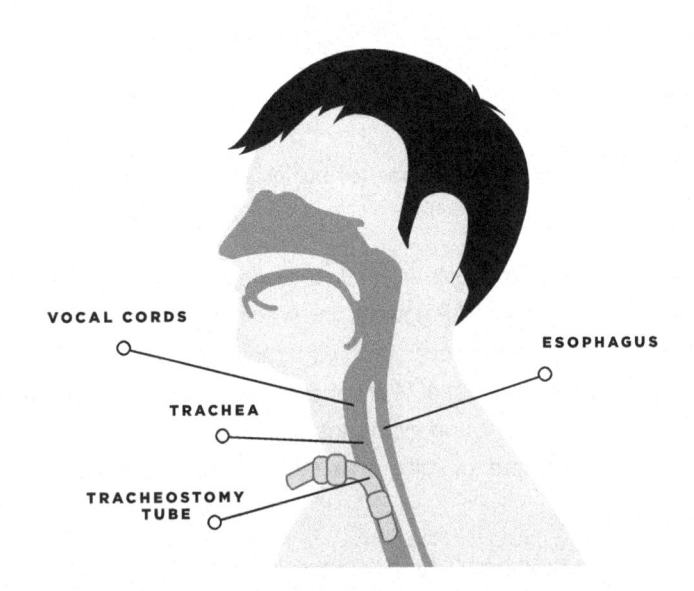

Figure 13. Bypassing the upper airway entirely can 'cure' OSA, but the other side effects and lifestyle issues make this a surgery of last resort.

Tongue Ties and Narrow Palates: Reshaping the Mouth

Palatal expansion is a common intervention for children whose SDB is due to a combination of a tethered tongue and a high narrow palate. While the process is more complicated for adults, often a parent looking for answers to a child's sleep breathing problems will realize that they themselves have the same physical problems and that they are also experiencing SDB because of them.

Eileen snored, but she was thin, active, and comparatively energetic, so her PCP never mentioned the possibility of UARS to her. When her son and nephew were both diagnosed with tongue-tie by SLPs and sent for revisions, she was confused. "But I can't do those things with my tongue either!"

In the office exam, we found a tethered tongue and a high, narrow palate that were contributing to her sleep breathing issues, and also some of her pronunciation issues when she tried to master foreign languages! After a tongue-tie release, an oral surgery, and six months of orthodontia, her palate is widened, her sinuses are improved, and she can properly position her tongue during sleep.

It's really common for patients to realize that they have a congenital issue when their kids are diagnosed with the same issue. Eileen is lucky that she got help before the cycle of weight gain, T2D, cardiovascular damage, and OSA kicked into gear.

Why Tongue Tie Affects Palates

A tongue-tie is a small bit of tissue that keeps the tongue from moving freely in the mouth. Tongue ties can affect infant feeding but also chewing and swallowing in toddlers and speech in older children. For centuries, the standard of care was to snip tongue ties at birth to prevent issues with nursing and later issues with speech and language. However, in the second half of the twentieth century, it became more common to take a wait and see approach. This is because some tongue ties loosen or break on their own, and bottle-fed babies can often feed well, even with a tongue-tie. So, a very safe, routine procedure became much rarer.

From a dental perspective, this shift in treatment philosophy was a disaster. In a healthy mouth, the tongue acts as a natural palate expander. It rests against the roof of the mouth during sleep, and the pressure flattens and widens the palate. This creates more room in the sinuses and makes room for the teeth.

A high narrow palate means that a child may have more difficulty with nasal breathing and resort to mouth breathing. They might have trouble moving food around their mouths. As their adult teeth come in, they may not have room for them all and, without palate expansion, may have to have healthy teeth pulled. While physicians may not see a compelling reason to snip all tongue ties, dentists, and speech pathologists recognize that the combination of tongue and palate issues can have life-long effects.

The process of expanding the palate normally begins in the womb. When a baby has a tongue-tie, they're born with a palate that is higher and narrower than usual. If the tongue-tie is released in the first few weeks of life, the tongue can rest in the proper position, and the palate can expand. But if it's left in place, the palate won't widen as the child grows.

The longer a child goes with a tongue tie, the less likely it is that tongue-tie release alone will restore the palate to a healthy place. Older children may need treatment to expand their palates so that they can master nasal breathing, speech sounds, and proper chewing. As a person grows, their palate becomes less amenable to expansion. We can fix palates in adults, but it's a more involved process.

Tongue Tie Revision—Ages and Solutions

The easiest time to revise a tongue tie is during the first few days of life. When a tongue tie is revised early in life, there's rarely any additional therapy or intervention needed. The revision involves holding the child still, releasing the tie with a laser or a pair of surgical scissors, and holding gauze to the wound for a few seconds. The child begins to feed well within moments after the tie is revised, and from this point on, the tongue and palate will develop normally.

Sometimes, no one mentions tongue-tie revision until the child is a toddler or preschooler. In these cases, it's usually a dentist or speech and language pathologist who finds the issue during an evaluation. For older children, the tongue-tie release can immediately improve nasal breathing, but therapy from an oral myofunctional therapist or a speech and language pathologist may be necessary to help improve drinking, eating, and speaking skills.

When a tongue-tie is revised for a toddler or preschooler, there's a chance that the child may need a palatal expander and braces later on. However, for many children, correcting the tongue tie prevents future problems.

When an older child or adult has a tongue-tie revision, they need therapy to improve speech, drinking, breathing, tongue position, and eating. They'll also need to undergo palate expansion and will probably need braces or a retainer. In general, with tongue ties, earlier revision is better. If you suspect your child has a tongue-tie, ask your dentist, pediatrician, or speech pathologist to check. Remember, tongue ties affect palate development. Ignoring one can cause a lifetime of sleep-disordered breathing and tooth and sinus issues.

Palatal Expansion in Children Before and During Puberty

For school-aged children, an unrevised tongue tie leads to a high, narrow palate. Even if the tie "broke" naturally in the preceding years, the child might not have developed the habit of placing the tongue high in the mouth. Without this habit, the palate won't expand, and it's hard to develop a habit of nasal breathing. Without nasal breathing, the nose can't do its job of warming, filtering, and moisturizing the air. Mouth breathing creates a cycle of irritation that leads to swollen tonsils and adenoids and UARS, SDB, or full-blown OSA in kids.

Rapid palatal expansion (RPE), also known as rapid maxillary expansion (RME), can widen the palate so that the tongue can rest on the roof of the mouth, the maxillary sinuses can expand properly, and the child can learn good nasal breathing habits. In children and teens, expanding the palate has been shown to improve or even cure UARS and other forms of SDB. It's even reversed treatment-resistant depression in teens because it treats the underlying cause of the depression—a restricted airway leading to disrupted sleep.

EXPANDING **THE PALATE**

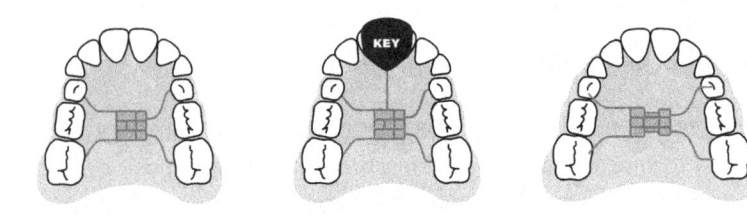

Figure 14. RPE uses an appliance to spread the palate over the course of several months.

In RPE, a dentist or orthodontist places an appliance in the upper jaw. The child must turn a key each night to expand the appliance and the palate bit by bit. This is possible because, in children, the palate is made of two separate bones. They don't fuse into a single piece until after the child is done growing. In children, using a palate expander to put pressure on the teeth will expand the palate.

In most cases, the rapid expansion process is complete in three to six months. After expansion, the child may need to wear a retainer or have braces for a while to help reposition the teeth. The palate expansion improves bite, leaves room for all the teeth, and, most importantly, opens up the airway so that the child can breathe. Some practices also offer children the chance to use a slower option where they only turn the key every other night instead of every night. This doubles the time in treatment but is an option for families who aren't comfortable with the more rapid pace.

Palate Expansion after Puberty

After puberty, palate expansion is more complicated. That's because once the bones have fused, it's harder to separate them and change their shape. For older teens and adults, the palate expansion process begins with either implants or surgery. In surgically assisted RPE, an oral surgeon makes cuts in the bone so that the palate can expand. Then, the expander is inserted so that it will put pressure on the bone and widen the palate. The patient grows new bone after the expansion process. In the implant process, implants inserted into the bone work with the palate expander to force the bones apart and the palate into the proper shape.

Once the palate has been expanded, braces or retainers can move the teeth into their permanent positions. The wide palate results in more open sinuses for better nasal breathing, better tongue position, and better sleep breathing. Many patients benefit from therapy with an OMT or SLP to improve their tongue positioning and motor skills after the expansion.

Implanted Device for OSA

Recently, the FDA has approved an implantable device for OSA. If your OSA is moderate to severe, you're not obese, and you can't tolerate PAP therapy, you may qualify for the device. It works by delivering a mild electric current to the muscles of your airway while you sleep. This prevents them from relaxing, collapsing, and cutting off your air supply.

The device is implanted during a two-hour out-patient surgery and calibrated a month later. It's battery-operated, and the batteries should last about a decade. While this is still a fairly new option for treating OSA, it's less invasive than UPPP and might be a good option for people who can't benefit from PAP or oral appliance therapy.

Diet and Exercise to Support Better Sleep

Diet and exercise are non-invasive and usually the first advice any medical professional will give you for *any problem at all*. So you may wonder why I'm putting it last, after all the other interventions for sleep issues. The answer is that to make healthy food choices and have the energy to exercise you need to be sleeping better.

Remember the changes that interrupted sleep makes to your brain and body? Not sleeping changes your cravings. It makes you tired and achy. It saps your will power and your ability to form new habits. So, while it's true that eating well, exercising, and losing weight will do great things for your sleep, you won't be able to make these life changes until you're getting some periods of good, unbroken rest.

But, once you *are* sleeping well, it's time to think about what to do with that newfound energy. And exercising, eating a balanced diet with lots of plant-based foods in the mix, and choosing healthy drinks over sugary drinks will let you feel better and help improve your sleep even more. So, like every other professional, I'm enthusiastically encouraging a balanced, healthy lifestyle because you deserve to live a long time and feel great while you're doing it.

The Take-Aways

- Everyone's body is different. Find out what *yours* needs for a good night's sleep.
- Everyone can benefit from creating a healthy bedroom environment and practicing good sleep hygiene.
- If underlying issues are causing your SDB, you need to address those to get the best possible outcomes.
- PAP devices and oral appliances are non-invasive, well-studied, common treatments for sleep issues.
- For children, surgery can be a first-line treatment for OSA. For adults, it is usually a treatment of last resort.

Try This

Go into each bedroom in your house and look around. What are three changes you can make in each one to create healthier sleep environments?

Things to Think About

- How can you and your family members improve your sleep hygiene?
- If you've tried one treatment and it hasn't worked, what will you try next?
- How often will you ask your care team about sleep issues and check in with them about your sleep?

12

On Your Way To Better Sleep

I hope that you now understand the magnitude of the sleeping crisis that America and your family face. Sleep is so important to every aspect of our lives, and our airways have an enormous impact on the quantity and quality of sleep we get. This is why I tell my patients that "Airway is Life." Without a functioning airway, you and your children fall prey to UARS and OSA. Sleep-disordered breathing is stealing your lives away, one day, one mood, and one memory at a time.

You also now understand who can help you treat these problems and how we can help you resolve them. This is important. Lost sleep is not inevitable. It is not some fact of modern life. It is a disease process, and the underlying condition is diagnosable and treatable. Even if you can't get your apneas and hypopneas down to zero, even if you can't stop all snoring or totally clear your airways, you can improve your condition.

Just like small sleep problems can spiral into bigger health problems, there's a snowball effect to sleep improvements. Improving your sleep even a little will help improve your life, your memory, your emotional control, and your willpower. And that little improvement will let you take other steps, which will eventually help improve your sleep even more. You and your family may be in crisis, but reading this book was the first step to getting out of that crisis. Now it's time to take the next steps to better sleep.

Step 1: Start Making Your Home Sleep-Friendly

As soon as you finish this book, you can make changes at home. In fact, you might have already started making changes once you realized how important sleep is. Make sure your family's bedrooms encourage sleep. Start trying to limit caffeine and blue light in the evening. Experiment to find your natural wakeup time, and try to get in bed nine hours before to give yourself plenty of time to sleep. If you have teens, do what you can to help them get enough sleep while respecting their circadian rhythms.

Step 2: Get Seen and Get Screened

If you, your partner, or one of your children show signs of sleep-disordered breathing, the first step is to get seen and get screened. Are you unsure who in your area is qualified to deal with sleep medicine? The American Academy of Sleep Medicine has an educational site at sleepeducation.org that can help you learn more about healthy sleep. The site includes a search tool that identifies sleep centers in your area. If you don't currently have a medical or dental provider, call the nearest sleep center and ask for recommendations.

Step 3: Make and Keep Those Appointments

I know you're busy. Specialist appointments take time out of a busy day, and they're yet one more thing to do when you're already stretched to the limit and totally exhausted. But these appointments are the first step towards feeling better. You *are* exhausted. We want you to have your energy back and to feel a decade (or more) younger. Make and keep those appointments, and get a treatment plan ASAP.

Step 4: Be Honest About Your Struggles

Thirty-two percent of people prescribed a CPAP, the first line of therapy for SDB in adults, don't use it. Many people only manage to use their CPAP for about half the night. If you've been prescribed a treatment that you can't use, your sleep-disordered breathing isn't being treated. Don't be afraid to ask your care team about other interventions like an APAP or an oral appliance. We want you to have a treatment plan that you can stick with, so you can get the benefits of good sleep.

If your child has had their tonsils and adenoids removed, but doesn't seem to be getting better, talk to someone. T&A helps many children, but it doesn't help all children, and your kid might be someone who needs a different approach.

Step 5: Be Willing to Get a Second Opinion

Sometimes, you hit a wall with treatment or a provider. It's OK to get a second opinion. Think of it like any other big healthcare commitment. If you take a kid in for braces and the orthodontist says, "We need to pull four healthy teeth," you would get consultations with other people to see if you could save the teeth, right?

This is true for sleep issues too. If one doctor tells you, "Well, there's nothing we can do," get a second opinion. Not everyone is trained in sleep medicine. Find a provider who is up to date in the field and willing to meet your family where they are.

Step 6: Become a Healthy Sleep Evangelist!

Once you've got your airways opened and your sleep issues resolved, you'll be feeling great. You'll finally have energy again; you can eat well and lose weight, learn new skills, and enjoy your family and friends. So, I want to ask one thing of you when you hit that point. Become a healthy sleep evangelist!

As I said before, sleep is one of the biggest health problems in our country today. And chances are friends and family are struggling. They're trying diet drinks and organizational plans and random cure-alls to try to get their energy back when the root issue is sleep-disordered breathing. They're losing years of their lives, and they have no one to let them know that the root cause of their issues is TREATABLE.

You can make a difference. You can get your friends and family healthy. You can save their lives. Share what you learned here with them. Share this book. Tell them about sleep and all it does. Get them screened, diagnosed, and treated. Spread the word about sleep, breathing, and living a long, healthy life.

Then, you can breathe easy and sleep well, knowing that you're doing all you can to keep everyone you love in good health.

Meghna Dassani DMD

Glossary of Sleep Science Terms

AHI	This stands for the apnea hypopnea index. It's a measure of the number of times your airway is fully or partially obstructed in an hour.
APAP	Automatic positive airway pressure machine. A machine that forces air through your airway as you sleep. It adjusts the force of the air to fit your needs depending on the stage of sleep and sleeping position.
Apnea	When your breathing temporarily stops during sleep.
ASPD	Advanced sleep phase disorder. A circadian rhythm disorder. People with ASPD like to fall asleep very early and wake up at 3:00 or 4:00 a.m. In general, this is more socially acceptable than DSPD since our society sees early risers as virtuous.
BiPAP	A machine that has two pressures, one for inhaling and one for exhaling, used to keep air flowing through the airways during sleep.
CBT	Cognitive behavioral therapy. A type of therapy that helps people understand what triggers their undesirable behaviors or thoughts and teaches them how to change those behaviors and thoughts by developing new physical and mental habits. This can successfully treat insomnia and improve sleep hygiene.
Circadian Rhythms	Our natural sleep-wake cycles; they're controlled by our clock genes and modified by environmental cues like sunlight or meal times. Things like our body temperature and hunger cues can be affected by them.
Cortisol	The stress hormone, it holds your body in "fight or flight" mode. It decreases during sleep.

CPAP	A continuous positive airway pressure machine. It has only one pressure, and is the same when you inhale, exhale, change position, or move through different sleep stages.
CSA	Central sleep apnea. When the brain itself causes sleep breathing to pause or stop.
Declarative Memory	Memory for facts like the name of a neighbor or a phone number.
DSPD	Delayed sleep phase disorder. A circadian rhythm disorder. Someone with DSPD is an extreme night owl and cannot get enough sleep if they have to live on a normal school or work schedule. However, these people are often fine if they can work the second or third shift.
EEG	Electroencephalogram. A machine that measures electrical activity in the brain. It can tell scientists what parts of the brain are used for different stages of sleep.
ENT	An ear, nose, and throat specialist. ENT's specialize in problems involving the upper airway.
Episodic Memory	Memories of experiences, including all five senses and feelings.
Ghrelin	The hormone that makes you hungry. It decreases while you sleep so that you don't need to eat overnight.
Growth Hormone	Released during sleep, it tells your body to grow and to heal the damage done to cells by being awake all day.
Hard Palate	The roof of your mouth. It's made of two bones that grow together during childhood. Behind it is the soft palate, which is made of muscle.
Homeostasis	From the Greek words meaning staying the same. It's your body's tendency to keep things like temperature and blood oxygen stable in the absence of stresses to the system.

Hypopnea	When your breathing is temporarily reduced but not totally stopped during sleep.
Leptin	The hormone that makes us feel full. It rises during sleep so that we don't crave food overnight.
Melatonin	A hormone that, among other things, causes us to get sleepy and stay asleep all night.
Microarousal	A brief awakening, only a few seconds long, that disrupts the sleep cycle but that the sleeper does not remember in the morning.
Neuroplasticity	Your brain's ability to rewire itself to adjust to your needs.
NREM	Non-rapid eye movement sleep. It's divided into three to four stages, including falling asleep, light sleep, and deep sleep (stages three and four). NREM is important for healing the body, learning and memory, and hormone regulation.
OAT	Oral appliance therapy. A way of treating SDB with a custom, removable oral appliance that keeps the airway open.
OMT	Oral myofunctional therapist. A physical and occupational therapist who specializes in issues of the mouth and throat. They can help with treating some forms of SDB.
OSA	Obstructive sleep apnea. When something is blocking your airways during sleep, causing you to periodically stop breathing.
Palate	The bone and muscle at the top of your mouth.
PAP	Positive airway pressure machine. One of several kinds of machines that use either a nose piece or a nose and mouth piece to force air through the airways during sleep in order to prevent apneas and hypopneas.
PLMS	Periodic limb movement syndrome. Apparently related to RLS, people who suffer from it thrash about during sleep, causing them to wake unrested.

Polysomnography	A sleep study where the sleep lab measures brain activity, muscle activity, breathing, and heart activity in order to determine how someone is sleeping and if they have any sleep disorders.
RDI	Respiratory disturbance index. More accurate than the AHI, it also takes into account the number of microarousals due to disordered breathing.
REM	Rapid eye movement sleep. This stage helps us with creativity, problem-solving, making connections between different parts of the brain, and social skills. During REM, our brain is as active as when we are awake, but our muscles are paralyzed to keep us from acting out what the brain is doing. This is a dream-heavy stage of sleep.
RERA	Respiratory effort related arousal. When a sleeper briefly awakes due to trouble breathing. These events are very brief, often only a second or two, so the sleeper won't remember them. However, they are enough to disrupt the work of sleep and cause complications.
RLS	Restless legs syndrome. A disorder where someone feels an unbearable urge to move their legs, especially as they fall asleep. It can interfere with falling and staying asleep and seems to be linked to a ferritin deficiency in many people.
RPE	Rapid palatal expansion. A system that uses a custom appliance on the roof of the mouth to treat high, narrow palates by spreading them out so that the mouth has room for the teeth and the nasal cavity is properly open.
SDB	Sleep-disordered breathing. Any issue with sleep breathing that affects the ability to fully rest and recuperate.
Sinus	Hollow cavities in the skull that help warm, filter, and humidify the air you breathe before it passes down the windpipe and into the lungs.

Sleep Cycle	How the body moves through all four stages of sleep. A sleep cycle lasts about ninety minutes, and they repeat throughout the night. As the night goes on, the composition of them shifts away from more slow-wave sleep and towards more REM sleep.
Sleep Hygiene	A set of behaviors and environmental changes that promote healthy sleep.
Slow Wave Sleep	The two deepest stages of NREM; they're characterized by waves of electricity pulsing rhythmically through the brain.
SLP	A speech and language pathologist. They can help with speech, feeding, and oral-motor issues. They are one of the kinds of specialists who often notice tongue tie, high palate, or a lack of nasal breathing.
Soft Palate	The muscle at the back of the roof of your mouth. It's essential for breathing, swallowing, and speaking. If it loses tone, it can block the airway during sleep.
Tongue Tie	When a band of tissue tethers the tongue to the floor of the mouth, reducing its ability to properly move or to reach the roof of the mouth. This can affect speech, eating, drinking, palate development, and sleep breathing.
T&A	Tonsillectomy and adenectomy. The first-line treatment for pediatric OSA; it's an outpatient surgery performed by an ENT to remove enlarged tonsils and adenoids.
UARS	Upper airway resistance syndrome. A milder form of SDB, often characterized by snoring, where extra effort is needed to breathe during sleep, but the airflow is never cut off. Untreated, it often progresses to full-blown OSA.
Upper Airway	The nose, sinuses, mouth, throat, and upper end of the trachea. It is the part of the body involved in sleep-disordered breathing.
Working Memory	The memory that lets you keep things ready as you finish complex tasks.

Further Reading

If you want to learn more about sleep, sleep breathing, hormones, and circadian rhythms, these are helpful resources written for general audiences.

Why We Sleep: Unlocking the Power of Sleep and Dreams by Matthew Walker. Penguin, 2018. One of America's leading sleep researchers explains the current state of the research. His descriptions of experiments and the effects of lost sleep are especially interesting.

Sleepyhead: The Neuroscience of a Good Night's Rest by Henry Nicholls. Basic Books, 2018. This book is written from the perspective of a man with narcolepsy trying to learn more about his condition and also about other sleep disorders. Since it focuses on disorders of sleep rather than healthy sleep, it gives a different viewpoint and covers different information than Walker's book.

"Governments Worldwide Consider Ditching Daylight Savings Time" in *Scientific American* on October 29, 2020. By Diana Kwon. (https://www.scientificamerican.com/article/governments-worldwide-consider-ditching-daylight-saving-time/) This article is useful for understanding how circadian rhythms and changes to our schedules can affect our ability to get a good night's sleep.

What to Expect During Polysomnography. A video by Children's Hospital of Orange County. (https://www.youtube.com/watch?v=WK-Dt-BZTqbg) While this video is aimed at children, it can also set adult minds at ease about sleep studies.

You and Your Hormones by the Society for Endocrinology (https://www.yourhormones.info/) This is a website designed to explain hormones to general audiences. It's a great place to learn more about the effects of sleep on hormones and how those hormones affect other systems of your body.

Sources

History of Sleep and Sleep Science

Barbera J. Sleep and dreaming in Greek and Roman philosophy. *Sleep Med.* 2008;9(8):906-910. doi:10.1016/j.sleep.2007.10.010

Dement W.C. The study of human sleep: a historical perspective. *Thorax* 1998;53:S2-S7.

Shepard JW Jr, Buysse DJ, Chesson AL Jr, et al. History of the development of sleep medicine in the United States. *J Clin Sleep Med.* 2005;1(1):61-82.

Sleep cycles

"Natural Patterns of Sleep." Harvard University Medical School Healthy Sleep website. (http://healthysleep.med.harvard.edu/healthy/science/what/sleep-patterns-rem-nrem)

"The Characteristics of Sleep" Harvard University Medical School Healthy Sleep Website. (http://healthysleep.med.harvard.edu/healthy/science/what/characteristics)

Sleep and hormones

Kim TW, Jeong JH, Hong SC. The impact of sleep and circadian disturbance on hormones and metabolism. *Int J Endocrinol.* 2015;2015:591729. doi:10.1155/2015/591729

Leproult R, Van Cauter E. Role of sleep and sleep loss in hormonal release and metabolism. *Endocr Dev.* 2010;17:11-21. doi:10.1159/000262524

Ruchała M, Bromińska B, Cyrańska-Chyrek E, Kuźnar-Kamińska B, Kostrzewska M, Batura-Gabryel H. Obstructive sleep apnea and hormones - a novel insight. *Arch Med Sci*. 2017;13(4):875-884. doi:10.5114/aoms.2016.61499

Spiegel K, Leproult R, L'Hermite-Balériaux M, Copinschi G, Penev P, Van Cauter E. Leptin Levels Are Dependent on Sleep Duration: Relationships with Sympathovagal Balance, Carbohydrate Regulation, Cortisol, and Thyrotropin, *The Journal of Clinical Endocrinology & Metabolism*, 2004 89(11): 5762–5771. doi:10.1210/jc.2004-1003

Van Cauter E, Plat L. Physiology of growth hormone secretion during sleep. *J Pediatr*. 1996;128(5 Pt 2):S32-S37. doi:10.1016/s0022-3476(96)70008-2

Anxiety and sleep

Ben Simon, E., Rossi, A., Harvey, A.G. *et al*. Overanxious and underslept. *Nat Hum Behav* **4**, 100–110 (2020). doi:10.1038/s41562-019-0754-8

Staner L. Sleep and anxiety disorders. *Dialogues Clin Neurosci*. 2003;5(3):249-258. doi:10.31887/DCNS.2003.5.3/lstaner

RLS

McManama Aukerman M, Aukerman D, Bayard M, Tudiver F, Thorp L, Bailey B. Exercise and Restless Legs Syndrome: A Randomized Controlled Trial. *The Journal of the American Board of Family Medicine* 2006, 19 (5) 487-493; DOI: 10.3122/jabfm.19.5.487

"Restless Legs Syndrome Fact Sheet", NINDS, Publication date May 2017. NIH Publication No. 17-4847 (*https://www.ninds.nih.gov/Disorders/Patient-Caregiver-Education/Fact-Sheets/Restless-Legs-Syndrome-Fact-Sheet*)

Restless Legs Syndrome (RLS) in Children and Adolescents. Cleveland Clinic website. (*https://my.clevelandclinic.org/health/ diseases/14309-restless-legs-syndrome-rls-in-children-and-adolescents*)

Circadian Rhythm Issues

Zee PC, Attarian H, Videnovic A. Circadian rhythm abnormalities. *Continuum (Minneap Minn)*. 2013;19(1 Sleep Disorders):132-147. doi:10.1212/01.CON.0000427209.21177.aa

Melatonin and ASD and ADHD

Braam W, Ehrhart F, Maas APHM, Smits MG, Curfs L. Low maternal melatonin level increases autism spectrum disorder risk in children. *Res Dev Disabil*. 2018;82:79-89. doi:10.1016/j.ridd.2018.02.017

Rossignol DA, Frye RE. Melatonin in autism spectrum disorders. *Curr Clin Pharmacol*. 2014;9(4):326-334. doi:10.2174/15748847113086 660072

Shomrat T, Nesher N. Updated View on the Relation of the Pineal Gland to Autism Spectrum Disorders. *Front. Endocrinol.*, 05 February 2019 | https://doi.org/10.3389/fendo.2019.00037

Sleep and Learning

Alhola P, Polo-Kantola P. Sleep deprivation: Impact on cognitive performance. *Neuropsychiatr Dis Treat*. 2007;3(5):553-567.

Bansal, D. Want to Learn a New Skill? Get Some Sleep. *University of California News Website*. (*https://www.universityofcalifornia.edu/ news/want-learn-new-skill-get-some-sleep*)

Bellesi M, Haswell JD, de Vivo L, Marshall W, Roseboom P, Tononi G, Cirelli C. Myelin modifications after chronic sleep loss in adolescent mice, *Sleep*, Volume 41, Issue 5, May 2018, zsy034, doi: 10.1093/sleep/zsy034

Chevalier N, Kurth S, Doucette MR, et al. Myelination Is Associated with Processing Speed in Early Childhood: Preliminary Insights. *PLoS One*. 2015;10(10):e0139897. Published 2015 Oct 6. doi:10.1371/journal.pone.0139897

College Students: Getting Enough Sleep is Vital for Academic Success. *AASM Website*. (https://aasm.org/college-students-getting-enough-sleep-is-vital-to-academic-success/)

de Vivo, L, Bellesi, M. The role of sleep and wakefulness in myelin plasticity. *Glia*. 2019; 67: 2142– 2152. *https://doi.org/10.1002/glia.23667*

Michigan State University. (2019, November 21). Science underestimated dangerous effects of sleep deprivation. *ScienceDaily*. Retrieved January 20, 2021 from www.sciencedaily.com/releases/2019/11/191121183923.htm

Okano, K., Kaczmarzyk, J.R., Dave, N. *et al.* Sleep quality, duration, and consistency are associated with better academic performance in college students. *npj Sci. Learn*. **4,** 16 (2019). https://doi.org/10.1038/s41539-019-0055-z

Ro, C. Why Sleep Should Be Every Student's Priority. *BBC Future.* (2018) **(https://www.bbc.com/future/article/20180815-why-sleep-should-be-every-students-priority)**

https://www.ncbi.nlm.nih.gov/pmc/articles/PMC4595421/

Sleep and Memory

Chai, Y., Fang, Z., Yang, F.N. *et al.* Two nights of recovery sleep restores hippocampal connectivity but not episodic memory after total sleep deprivation. *Sci Rep* **10,** 8774 (2020). https://doi.org/10.1038/s41598-020-65086-x

Diekelmann, S., Born, J. The memory function of sleep. *Nat Rev Neurosci* **11,** 114–126 (2010). *https://doi.org/10.1038/nrn2762*

Lewine H. Too Little Sleep, and Too Much, Affect Memory. *Harvard Health Blog*. (https://www.health.harvard.edu/blog/little-sleep-much-affect-memory-201405027136)

Michigan State University. (2018, October 2). How sleep deprivation hinders memory. *ScienceDaily*. Retrieved January 20, 2021 from *www.sciencedaily.com/releases/2018/10/181002114027.htm*

Tantawy AO, Tallawy HN, Farghaly HR, Farghaly WM, Hussein AS. Impact of nocturnal sleep deprivation on declarative memory retrieval in students at an orphanage: a psychoneuroradiological study. *Neuropsychiatr Dis Treat*. 2013;9:403-408. doi:10.2147/NDT.S38905

Sleep and Emotional Control

Cohut M. This is How Sleep Loss Alters Emotional Perception. *Medical News Today*. (https://www.medicalnewstoday.com/articles/324937)

Harrington MO, Ashton JE, Sankarasubramanian S, Anderson MC, Cairney SA. Losing Control: Sleep Deprivation Impairs the Suppression of Unwanted Thoughts. *Clinical Psychological Science*. October 2020. doi:*10.1177/2167702620951511*

Saghir Z, Syeda JN, Muhammad AS, Balla Abdalla TH. The Amygdala, Sleep Debt, Sleep Deprivation, and the Emotion of Anger: A Possible Connection?. *Cureus*. 2018;10(7):e2912. Published 2018 Jul 2. doi:10.7759/cureus.2912

Vandekerckhove M, Wang YL. Emotion, emotion regulation and sleep: An intimate relationship. *AIMS Neurosci*. 2017;5(1):1-17. Published 2017 Dec 1. doi:10.3934/Neuroscience.2018.1.1

https://journals.sagepub.com/doi/full/10.1177/2167702620951511

Hamzelou J. Why Lack of Sleep Makes Us Emotionally Distracted by Everything. *New Scientist*. 25 Sep 2015. (*https://www.newscientist.com/article/dn28236-why-lack-of-sleep-makes-us-emotionally-distracted-by-everything/*)

Sleep and Mental Illness

Miller S. Lack of Sleep May Be a Cause, Not a Symptom, of Mental Health Conditions. *Livescience Website*. 6 Sep 2017. (https://www.livescience.com/60329-online-insomnia-therapy-mental-health-symptoms.html)

Medical College of Georgia at Augusta University. "Obstructive sleep apnea may be one reason depression treatment doesn't work." ScienceDaily. ScienceDaily, 23 July 2019. <www.sciencedaily.com/releases/2019/07/190723104041.htm>.

Sleep and Mental Health: Sleep Deprivation Can Affect Your Mental Health. *Harvard Mental Health Letter*. 18 Mar 2019. (https://www.health.harvard.edu/newsletter_article/sleep-and-mental-health)

Swaminathan N. Can Lack of Sleep Cause Psychiatric Disorders? *Scientific American*. 23 Oct 2007. (https://www.scientificamerican.com/article/can-a-lack-of-sleep-cause/)

Social Life and Sleep

Anwar Y. Poor Sleep Can Literally Kill Your Social Life. *University of California News Website*. (https://www.universityofcalifornia.edu/news/poor-sleep-can-literally-kill-your-social-life)

Christian M, Ellis A. Examining the Effects of Sleep Deprivation on Workplace Deviance: A Self-Regulatory Perspective. (2011) *AMJ*, **54**, 913–934, *https://doi.org/10.5465/amj.2010.0179*

Holding, B.C., Sundelin, T., Lekander, M. et al. Sleep deprivation and its effects on communication during individual and collaborative tasks. *Sci Rep* **9**, 3131 (2019). *https://doi.org/10.1038/s41598-019-39271-6*

Sleep and Habits

Chen J, Liang J, Lin X, Zhang Y, Zhang Y, Lu L, Shi J. Sleep Deprivation Promotes Habitual Control over Goal-Directed Control: Behavioral and Neuroimaging Evidence. *Journal of Neuroscience* 6 December 2017, 37 (49) 11979-11992; DOI: 10.1523/JNEUROSCI.1612-17.2017

Dartmouth College. How the Brain Forms Habits. *Neuroscience News Website.* (https://neurosciencenews.com/habits-brain-15805/)

Massachusetts Institute of Technology. "Distinctive brain pattern helps habits form: Study identifies neurons that fire at the beginning and end of a behavior as it becomes a habit." ScienceDaily. ScienceDaily, 8 February 2018. <www.sciencedaily.com/releases/2018/02/180208120923.htm>.

Pilcher J, Morris D, Donnelly J, Feigl H. Interactions between sleep habits and self-control. *Frontiers in Human Neuroscience* (2019) 9:284 doi:10.3389/fnhum.2015.00284

Vyazovskiy V, Walton M, Peirson S, Bannerman D. Sleep homeostasis, habits and habituation. *Current Opinion in Neurobiology.* Volume 44, 2017, Pages 202-211,ISSN 0959-4388,https://doi.org/10.1016/j.conb.2017.05.002.

Sleep and Eating

Greer SM, Goldstein AN, Walker MP. The impact of sleep deprivation on food desire in the human brain. *Nat Commun.* 2013;4:2259. doi:10.1038/ncomms3259

Hanlon EC, Tasali E, Leproult R, et al. Sleep Restriction Enhances the Daily Rhythm of Circulating Levels of Endocannabinoid 2-Arachidonoylglycerol. *Sleep.* 2016;39(3):653-664. Published 2016 Mar 1. doi:10.5665/sleep.5546

Henst, RHP, Pienaar, PR, Roden, LC, Rae, DE. The effects of sleep extension on cardiometabolic risk factors: A systematic review. *J Sleep Res.* 2019; 28:e12865. https://doi.org/10.1111/jsr.12865

Sleep and Pain

Finan PH, Goodin BR, Smith MT. The association of sleep and pain: an update and a path forward. *J Pain*. 2013;14(12):1539-1552. doi:10.1016/j.jpain.2013.08.007

Society for Neuroscience. "Poor sleep at night, more pain the next day." ScienceDaily. ScienceDaily, 29 January 2019. <www.sciencedaily.com/releases/2019/01/190129093714.htm>.

Sleep and the Immune system

Hsiao YH, Chen YT, Tseng CM, Wu LA, Lin WC, MD, Su V, et al. Sleep Disorders and Increased Risk of Autoimmune Diseases in Individuals without Sleep Apnea, *Sleep*, Volume 38, Issue 4, 1 April 2015, Pages 581–586, *https://doi.org/10.5665/sleep.4574*

Palma BD, Gabriel A Jr, Colugnati FA, Tufik S. Effects of sleep deprivation on the development of autoimmune disease in an experimental model of systemic lupus erythematosus. *Am J Physiol Regul Integr Comp Physiol*. 2006;291(5):R1527-R1532. doi:10.1152/ajpregu.00186.2006

University of Washington Health Sciences/UW Medicine. "Chronic sleep deprivation suppresses immune system: Study one of first conducted outside of sleep lab." ScienceDaily. ScienceDaily, 27 January 2017. <www.sciencedaily.com/releases/2017/01/170127113010.htm>.

Alcoholism and OSA

Alcoholism: Clinical & Experimental Research. "Recovering Alcoholics With Poor Sleep Perceptions Will Likely Relapse." ScienceDaily. ScienceDaily, 27 November 2006. <www.sciencedaily.com/releases/2006/11/061127141315.htm>.

Brooks, A.T., Kazmi, N., Yang, L. *et al.* Sleep-Related Cognitive/Behavioral Predictors of Sleep Quality and Relapse in Individuals with Alcohol Use Disorder. *Int.J. Behav. Med.* (2020). https://doi.org/10.1007/s12529-020-09901-9

Brower K, Aldrich M, Robinson E, Zucker R, Greden J.Insomnia, Self-Medication, and Relapse to Alcoholism. *The American journal of psychiatry.* 158. Doi:10.1176/appi.ajp.158.3.399

Gestational OSA

Dominguez JE, Street L, Louis J. Management of Obstructive Sleep Apnea in Pregnancy. *Obstet Gynecol Clin North Am.* 2018;45(2):233-247. doi:10.1016/j.ogc.2018.01.001

Street LM, Aschenbrenner CA, Houle TT, Pinyan CW, Eisenach JC. Gestational Obstructive Sleep Apnea: Biomarker Screening Models and Lack of Postpartum Resolution. *J Clin Sleep Med.* 2018;14(4):549-555. Published 2018 Apr 15. doi:10.5664/jcsm.7042

OSA and Alzheimers

Andrade AG, Bubu OM, Varga AW, Osorio RS. The Relationship between Obstructive Sleep Apnea and Alzheimer's Disease. *J Alzheimers Dis.* 2018;64(s1):S255-S270. doi:10.3233/JAD-179936

Polsek D, Gildeh N, Cash D, et al. Obstructive sleep apnoea and Alzheimer's disease: In search of shared pathomechanisms. *Neurosci Biobehav Rev.* 2018;86:142-149. doi:10.1016/j.neubiorev.2017.12.004

RMIT University. "Identical signs of brain damage in sleep apnea and Alzheimer's." ScienceDaily. ScienceDaily, 28 September 2020. <www.sciencedaily.com/releases/2020/09/200928103416.htm>.

Sleep Apnea in Later Life More Than Doubles Subsequent Alzheimer's Disease Risk. *Neurology Reviews.* 2016 August;24(8):20 (https://www.mdedge.com/neurology/article/110883/sleep-medicine/sleep-apnea-later-life-more-doubles-subsequent-alzheimers?sso=true)

Diabetes and OSA

Doumit J and Prasad B. Sleep Apnea in Type 2 Diabetes. *Diabetes Spectrum* 2016 Feb; 29(1): 14-19. https://doi.org/10.2337/diaspect.29.1.14

Lecube A, Sampol G, Hernández C, Romero O, Ciudin A, et al. (2015) Characterization of Sleep Breathing Pattern in Patients with Type 2 Diabetes: Sweet Sleep Study. PLOS ONE 10(3): e0119073. https://doi.org/10.1371/journal.pone.0119073

Reichmuth KJ, Austin D, Skatrud JB, Young T. Association of sleep apnea and type II diabetes: a population-based study. *Am J Respir Crit Care Med*. 2005;172(12):1590-1595. doi:10.1164/rccm.200504-637OC

Reutrakul S, Mokhlesi B. Obstructive Sleep Apnea and Diabetes: A State of the Art Review. *Chest*. 2017;152(5):1070-1086. doi:10.1016/j.chest.2017.05.009

Cardiac Arrhythmia and OSA

Hersi AS. Obstructive sleep apnea and cardiac arrhythmias. *Ann Thorac Med*. 2010;5(1):10-17. doi:10.4103/1817-1737.58954

Patel AR, Patel AR, Singh S, Singh S, Khawaja I. The Association Between Obstructive Sleep Apnea and Arrhythmias. *Cureus*. 2019;11(4):e4429. Published 2019 Apr 10. doi:10.7759/cureus.4429

Wickramasinghe H. Cardiovascular Disease in Obstructive Sleep Apnea. *Medscape Website. (https://www.medscape.com/answers/295807-53550/what-is-the-association-between-obstructive-sleep-apnea-osa-and-cardiac-arrhythmias)*

SDB and Obesity

Leinum CJ, Dopp JM, Morgan BJ. Sleep-disordered breathing and obesity: pathophysiology, complications, and treatment. *Nutr Clin Pract*. 2009;24(6):675-687. doi:10.1177/0884533609351532

Ryan S, Crinion SJ, McNicholas WT. Obesity and sleep-disordered breathing—when two 'bad guys' meet, *QJM: An International Journal of Medicine*, Volume 107, Issue 12, December 2014, Pages 949–954, *https://doi.org/10.1093/qjmed/hcu029https://www.ncbi.nlm.nih.gov/pmc/articles/PMC4344922/*

SDB and Cancer

Martínez-García MA, Campos-Rodríguez F, Farré R. Sleep apnoea and cancer: current insights and future perspectives. *European Respiratory Journal* 2012 40: 1315-1317; DOI: 10.1183/09031936.00127912

Paddock C. Cancer More Common in Females with Severe Sleep Apnea. *Medical News Today Website*. (*https://www.medicalnewstoday.com/articles/326116*)

Sillah A, Watson NF, Gozal D, Phipps AI. Obstructive sleep apnea severity and subsequent risk for cancer incidence. *Prev Med Rep*. 2019;15:100886. Published 2019 May 2. doi:10.1016/j.pmedr.2019.100886

Some Cancers May Be Related to Sleep Apnea. *American Thoracic Society Website*. (*https://www.thoracic.org/about/newsroom/press-releases/journal/2020/some-cancers-may-be-related-to-sleep-apnea.php*)

SDB and Hypertension

Dopp JM, Reichmuth KJ, Morgan BJ. Obstructive sleep apnea and hypertension: mechanisms, evaluation, and management. *Curr Hypertens Rep*. 2007;9(6):529-534. doi:10.1007/s11906-007-0095-2

Lee C-H, Kang K-T, Chiu S-N, et al. *Association of adenotonsillectomy with blood pressure among hypertensive and nonhypertensive children with obstructive sleep apnea [published online February 15, 2018]. JAMA Otolaryngol Head Neck Surg.* doi:10.1001/jamaoto.2017.3127

Marcus CL, Greene MG, Carroll JL. Blood pressure in children with obstructive sleep apnea. *Am J Respir Crit Care Med.* 1998;157(4 Pt 1):1098-1103. doi:10.1164/ajrccm.157.4.9704080

Phillips CL, O'Driscoll DM. Hypertension and obstructive sleep apnea. *Nat Sci Sleep.* 2013;5:43-52. Published 2013 May 10. doi:10.2147/NSS.S34841

Sharabi Y, Scope A, Chorney N, Grotto I, Dagan Y. Diastolic blood pressure is the first to rise in association with early subclinical obstructive sleep apnea: lessons from periodic examination screening. *Am J Hypertens.* 2003;16(3):236-239. doi:10.1016/s0895-7061(02)03250-8

SBD and autoimmune diseases

Chen WS, Chang YS, Chang CC, et al. Management and Risk Reduction of Rheumatoid Arthritis in Individuals with Obstructive Sleep Apnea: A Nationwide Population-Based Study in Taiwan. *Sleep.* 2016;39(10):1883-1890. Published 2016 Oct 1. doi:10.5665/sleep.6174

Kang JH, Lin HC. Obstructive sleep apnea and the risk of autoimmune diseases: a longitudinal population-based study. *Sleep Med.* 2012;13(6):583-588. doi:10.1016/j.sleep.2012.03.002

Mann A. Study Explores Sleep Apnea, Autoimmune Disease Link. *University of Georgia News Website. (https://news.uga.edu/study-sleep-apnea-autoimmune-disease/)*

Phillips B, Wang Y, Ambati S, Ma P, Meagher R. Airways therapy of obstructive sleep apnea dramatically improves aberrant levels of soluble cytokines involved in autoimmune disease. *Clinical Immunology*, 2020. Doi:10.1016/j.clim.2020.108601

OSA and atherosclerosis

Floras J. Hypertension, Sleep Apnea, and Atherosclerosis. *Hypertension.* 2009;53:1–3. doi:10.1161/HYPERTENSIONAHA.108.123711

Lévy P, Pépin JL, Arnaud C, Baguet JP, Dematteis M, Mach F. Obstructive sleep apnea and atherosclerosis. *Prog Cardiovasc Dis.* 2009;51(5):400-410. doi:10.1016/j.pcad.2008.03.001

Lui MM, Sau-Man M. OSA and atherosclerosis. *J Thorac Dis.* 2012;4(2):164-172. doi:10.3978/j.issn.2072-1439.2012.01.06

Wickramasinghe H. What is the association between atherosclerosis and obstructive sleep apnea (OSA)? *Medscape Website. (https://www.medscape.com/answers/295807-53548/what-is-the-association-between-atherosclerosis-and-obstructive-sleep-apnea-osa)*

Heart Failure and SDB

Gavadia M. What is the Relationship Between OSA, Cardiovascular Disease. *AJMC Website. (https://www.ajmc.com/view/what-is-the-relationship-between-osa-cardiovascular-disease)*

Khattak HK, Hayat F, Pamboukian SV, Hahn HS, Schwartz BP, Stein PK. Obstructive Sleep Apnea in Heart Failure: Review of Prevalence, Treatment with Continuous Positive Airway Pressure, and Prognosis. *Tex Heart Inst J.* 2018;45(3):151-161. Published 2018 Jun 1. doi:10.14503/THIJ-15-5678

Specific Sleep Apnea Subtype Increases Heart Failure Risk. *Pulmonology Advisor Website. (https://www.pulmonologyadvisor.com/home/topics/obstructive-sleep-apnea-osa/specific-sleep-apnea-subtype-increases-heart-failure-risk/)*

OSA Stroke

Chan W, Coutts SB, Hanly P. Sleep apnea in patients with transient ischemic attack and minor stroke: opportunity for risk reduction of recurrent stroke?. *Stroke.* 2010;41(12):2973-2975. doi:10.1161/STROKEAHA.110.596759

Jehan S, Farag M, Zizi F, et al. Obstructive sleep apnea and stroke. *Sleep Med Disord.* 2018;2(5):120-125.

Gavadia, M. How Can Snoring Patterns Help Predict Risk of Stroke in High-Risk Patients With Obstructive Sleep Apnea? *AJMC Website.* (https://www.ajmc.com/view/how-can-snoring-patterns-help-predict-risk-of-stroke-in-highrisk-patients-with-obstructive-sleep-apnea)

Obstructive Sleep Apnea and Stroke. *AAST Website.* (https://www.aastweb.org/blog/obstructive-sleep-apnea-and-stroke)

Early Death and OSA

Franklin K, Linberg E. Obstructive sleep apnea is a common disorder in the population—a review on the epidemiology of sleep apnea. *Journal of Thoracic Disease* 7:8

Obstructive Sleep Apnea Raises Risk of Sudden Death, Mayo Clinic Finds. *Mayo Clinic Website.* (https://newsnetwork.mayoclinic.org/discussion/obstructive-sleep-apnea-raises-risk-of-sudden-cardiac-death-mayo-clinic-finds/)

Sleep Apnea Surgery Patients at Risk of Cardiac Events, Including Death. *Same Day Surgery Online.* (https://www.reliasmedia.com/articles/144558-sleep-apnea-surgery-patients-at-risk-of-cardiac-events-including-death)

Study Shows That People with Sleep Apnea Have a Higher Risk of Death. *AASM Website* (https://aasm.org/study-shows-that-people-with-sleep-apnea-have-a-high-risk-of-death/)

Wickramasinghe H. What is the mortality rate for sleep apnea (OSA)? *Medscape Website*. (https://www.medscape.com/answers/295807-53497/what-is-the-mortality-rate-for-sleep-apnea-osa)

Wong M. 5 Facts That Make Patients with OSA More at Risk for Death. *Physician-Patient Alliance for Health and Safety Website*. (http://ppahs.org/2018/03/5-facts-that-makes-patients-with-obstructive-sleep-apnea-more-at-risk-for-death/)

Sleep and Failure at School and Work

American Academy of Sleep Medicine. "Sleep apnea in children and teens to linked to lower academic grades." ScienceDaily. ScienceDaily, 8 June 2010. <www.sciencedaily.com/releases/2010/06/100608091854.htm>.

American Academy of Sleep Medicine. Adults with Sleep Apnea More Likely to Experience Involuntary Job Loss. *AASM Website*. (https://aasm.org/sleep-apnea-job-loss/)

Bonuck K, Rao T, Xu L. Pediatric sleep disorders and special educational need at 8 years: a population-based cohort study. *Pediatrics*. 2012;130(4):634-642. doi:10.1542/peds.2012-0392

Goyal A, Pakhare AP, Bhatt GC, Choudhary B, Patil R. Association of pediatric obstructive sleep apnea with poor academic performance: A school-based study from India. *Lung India*. 2018;35(2):132-136. doi:10.4103/lungindia.lungindia_218_17

Ikeda FH, Campos-Horta P, Bruscato W, Dolci J. Intellectual and school performance evaluation of children submitted to tonsillectomy and adenotonsillectomy before and after surgery. *Brazilian Journal of Otorhinolaryngology*. Volume 78, Issue 4, July–August 2012, Pages 17-23

Jennum P, Ibsen R, Kjellberg J. Social consequences of sleep disordered breathing on patients and their partners: a controlled national study. *European Respiratory Journal* 2014 43: 134-144; DOI: 10.1183/09031936.00169212

Omachi TA, Claman DM, Blanc PD, Eisner MD. Obstructive sleep apnea: a risk factor for work disability. *Sleep*. 2009;32(6):791-798. doi:10.1093/sleep/32.6.791

SWANSON, L.M., ARNEDT, J.T., ROSEKIND, M.R., BELENKY, G., BALKIN, T.J. and DRAKE, C. (2011), Sleep disorders and work performance: findings from the 2008 National Sleep Foundation Sleep in America poll. Journal of Sleep Research, 20: 487-494. *https://doi.org/10.1111/j.1365-2869.2010.00890.x*

OSA and Mental Health

Bishop TM, Ashrafioun L, Pigeon WR. The Association Between Sleep Apnea and Suicidal Thought and Behavior: An Analysis of National Survey Data. *J Clin Psychiatry*. 2018;79(1):17m11480. doi:10.4088/JCP.17m11480

Krahn LE, Miller BW, Bergstrom LR. Rapid resolution of intense suicidal ideation after treatment of severe obstructive sleep apnea. *J Clin Sleep Med*. 2008;4(1):64-65.

Sandoiu A. What is the Link Between Sleep Apnea and Depression? *Medical News Today Website. (https://www.medicalnewstoday.com/articles/325839)*

Sleep screening tools

https://qxmd.com/calculate/calculator_85/epworth-sleepiness-scale

https://qxmd.com/calculate/calculator_531/stop-bang-score-for-obstructive-sleep-apnea

https://qxmd.com/calculate/calculator_603/pittsburgh-sleep-quality-index-psqi

https://www.usa.philips.com/c-dam/b2bhc/master/whitepapers/sleep-therapy/1040664_BerlinQNCRForms.pdf

CBT for sleep issues

Anderson KN. Insomnia and cognitive behavioural therapy-how to assess your patient and why it should be a standard part of care. *J Thorac Dis*. 2018;10(Suppl 1):S94-S102. doi:10.21037/jtd.2018.01.35

Insomnia Treatment: Cognitive Behavioral Therapy Instead Of Sleeping Pills. *Mayo Clinic. (https://www.mayoclinic.org/diseases-conditions/insomnia/in-depth/insomnia-treatment/art-20046677)*

Sweetman A, Lack L, Catcheside PG, et al. Cognitive and behavioral therapy for insomnia increases the use of continuous positive airway pressure therapy in obstructive sleep apnea participants with comorbid insomnia: a randomized clinical trial. Sleep. 2019;42(12):zsz178. doi:10.1093/sleep/zsz178

Sweetman A, Lack L, Catcheside PG, et al. Cognitive behavioural therapy for insomnia reduces sleep apnoea severity: a randomised controlled trial. *ERJ Open Research* Apr 2020, 6 (2) 00161-2020; DOI: 10.1183/23120541.00161-2020

Melatonin and Sleep

Gagnon K, Godbout R. Melatonin and Comorbidities in Children with Autism Spectrum Disorder. *Curr Dev Disord Rep*. 2018;5(3):197-206. doi:10.1007/s40474-018-0147-0

Hardeland R. Neurobiology, pathophysiology, and treatment of melatonin deficiency and dysfunction. *ScientificWorldJournal*. 2012;2012:640389. doi:10.1100/2012/640389

Allergy Meds and SDB

Brouilette R, Manoukian J, Ducharme F, Oudjhane K, et al. Efficacy of fluticasone nasal spray for pediatric obstructive sleep apnea. July 2001. *Journal of Pediatrics* 138(6):838-44 DOI: 10.1067/mpd.2001.114474

Tam YY, Shao IH, Wu CC, Hsieh ML. The impact of intranasal fluticasone on patients with obstructive sleep apnea: a prospective study [published online ahead of print, 2019 Aug 31]. Braz J Otorhinolaryngol. 2019;S1808-8694(19)30092-8. doi:10.1016/j.bjorl.2019.07.007

PAP Therapy

Continuous Positive Airway Pressure for Adults with Sleep Apnea. *American Thoracic Society Website. (https://www.thoracic.org/patients/patient-resources/resources/cpap-for-osa.pdf)*

OAT

Jayesh SR, Bhat WM. Mandibular advancement device for obstructive sleep apnea: An overview. *J Pharm Bioallied Sci*. 2015;7(Suppl 1):S223-S225. doi:10.4103/0975-7406.155915

Joshi, A. Oral Appliances in Snoring and Obstructive Sleep Apnea. *Medscape Website. (https://emedicine.medscape.com/article/869831-overview)*

Marklund M, Johan Verbraecken J, Randerath W. Non-CPAP therapies in obstructive sleep apnoea: mandibular advancement device therapy. *European Respiratory Journal* 2012 39: 1241-1247; DOI: 10.1183/09031936.00144711

RPE

Detailleur V, Cadenas de Llano-Pérula M, Buyse B, Verdonck A, Politis C, et al. (2017) Are Sleep Disordered Breathing Symptoms and Maxillary Expansion Correlated? A Prospective Evaluation Study. *J Sleep Disor: Treat Care* 6:1. doi: 10.4172/2325-9639.1000186

Miller P, Iyer M, Gold AR. Treatment resistant adolescent depression with upper airway resistance syndrome treated with rapid palatal expansion: a case report. *J Med Case Rep*. 2012;6:415. Published 2012 Dec 4. doi:10.1186/1752-1947-6-415

Villa MP, Rizzoli A, Rabasco J, et al. Rapid maxillary expansion outcomes in treatment of obstructive sleep apnea in children. *Sleep Med*. 2015;16(6):709-716. doi:10.1016/j.sleep.2014.11.019

https://dentalsleeppractice.com/articles/treating-sleep-disorders-with-oral-appliances/

OMT

Karon A. Oropharyngeal exercises significantly cuts snoring. *MD Edge News Website*.

(https://www.mdedge.com/chestphysician/article/102780/sleep-medicine/oropharyngeal-exercises-significantly-cuts-snoring?sso=true)

Implanted stimulation

Boon M, Huntley C, Steffen A, et al. Upper Airway Stimulation for Obstructive Sleep Apnea: Results from the ADHERE Registry. *Otolaryngol Head Neck Surg*. 2018;159(2):379-385. doi:10.1177/0194599818764896